A Theory-based Approach to Art Therapy

Art therapy literature is often based either on practice in a specific setting, art material or population, or if taking a more theoretical focus, on illustrative case studies. This book provides a theory-based approach to research, teaching, and practising art therapy, including verbal and art-based techniques, settings, art processes and analyses, and the principles of supervision, evaluation, and research. It also offers an overview and discussion of how the different orientations of psychological and social theories are interpreted and implemented by art therapy.

The book provides an integrative perspective that anchors methodology within a rigorous theoretical background. Focusing on three sub-groups of dynamic, humanistic and systemic-social theories, each chapter outlines the central concepts of varying sub-theories within a general heading, and their interpretation from an art therapy perspective. Ephrat Huss explores the respective and shifting roles of art, client, and therapist through each theory, demonstrating the practical implications for creating a coherent intervention that informs all parts of the setting, therapy, client evaluation, and supervision.

A Theory-based Approach to Art Therapy draws on the latest research in the field and will be a valuable text for art therapy theorists, educators, students and researchers, as well as for other social practitioners interested in understanding how to integrate art into their practice.

Ephrat Huss is Senior Lecturer at Ben-Gurion University, Israel, and Chair of the Arts in Social Practice MA specialization. Before this, she worked for many years as a supervising art therapist, family therapist, and social worker before turning to research, and still strongly believes in the connection between theory and practice.

Explorations in Mental Health series

Books in this series:

A Theory-based Approach to Art Therapy

Implications for teaching, research, and practice

Ephrat Huss

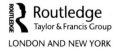

Routledge
Taylor & Francis Group

LONDON AND NEW YORK

First published 2015
by Routledge
27 Church Road, Hove, East Sussex, BN3 2FA

and by Routledge
711 Third Avenue, New York, NY 10017

Routledge is an imprint of the Taylor and Francis Group, an informa business

British Library Cataloguing in Publication Data
A catalogue record for this book is available from the British Library

Library of Congress Cataloguing in Publication data
Huss, Ephrat, author.
   A theory-based approach to art therapy : implications for teaching, research and practice / Ephrat Huss.
      p. ; cm.
   Includes bibliographical references and index.
   I. Title.
   [DNLM: 1. Art Therapy. 2. Psychological Theory. WM 450.5.A8]
   RC489.A7
   616.89'1656–dc23   2014042487

ISBN: 978-0-415-72544-6 (hbk)
ISBN: 978-1-315-85681-0 (ebk)

Typeset in Bembo
by Out of House Publishing

Contents

List of figures

List of tables

Introduction

In general, art therapists and all social practitioners tend to be bored by theory: indeed, theory sounds like a nice pursuit for academics and writers, but social practitioners with a client appearing at the door on the hour don't have time to delve into theoretical issues. Theory and practice are often experienced as two disconnected areas: 'practice knowledge' is different from theoretical knowledge. In art therapy specifically, theory is therefore often viewed with suspicion as something that is external to art therapy, coming from psychology, from art, or from a place that distances art from therapy, or therapy from art. There is much debate around the relative power of 'art' versus 'therapy'; as in the 'art as psychotherapy' versus 'art as therapy' debate, which becomes an effort to prove to the holders of psychological theory that art provides therapeutic results. Conversely, the other direction is to prove to the art sides that art is in itself healing: sometimes this includes sweeping declarations that art is above or beyond, or does not need 'theory'.

The claim of this book is that art therapy must base itself clearly within theoretical frames. While theory is never absolute truth, it is a vital and evolving set of ideas about how to make the pain of living in the world more bearable. It is a set of assumptions about what is a problem, and what is a solution, at a given place and time in history. Each psychological theory – dynamic, object relations, ego psychology, humanistic, existential, gestalt, narrative mind-body, cognitive behaviour therapy (CBT), systemic empowerment, social change, and cultural theories, to name a few – has a conception of what is a problem, what is a solution, and what is the role of art in relation to the theory of therapy. This provides a base for understanding the relationship of art to therapy, and for understanding how to use art within therapy. Theory defines the role of art within art therapy as inherent, rather than as randomly based on the techniques the therapist likes most, or what worked best with the last client, or on general 'recipes' according to generalizations about the client type, or the problem type. A theoretical understanding of how art is conceptualized within each theory enables it to be used coherently and professionally, as well as in the most flexible manner, because the core assumptions of the theory can be translated in many ways, while still creating unity between the therapeutic contract, setting, evaluation, supervision, and art use, that all correlate through the basic assumptions of the theory. This enables the art therapist to be more professional, not because they are more insightful or sensitive than the client, or because art is inherently healing (otherwise all artists would be healthy), but because they are professionals following a theoretical frame that makes sense of the client's problem and solution, and of how art can help reach this solution. This book will show that, paradoxically, taking time to weave theory more inherently into art therapy is not limiting to creativity, but rather enables a broader and more flexible base for art within therapy.

There are many books within art therapy that describe different art activities, often directed for use with specific populations (Abraham, 2001; Arrington, 2001; Buchalter, 2009; Cary and Rubin, 2006; Case and Daley, 1990; Docktor, 1994; Dubowski and Evans, 2001; Gil, 2006; Kalmanowitz and Lloyd, 2005; Liebmann, 1994; Linesch 1993; Magniant and Freeman, 2004; Malchiodi, 1997, 1999, 2007; Meekums, 2000; Meijer-Degen, 2006; Miller, 1996; Moschino, 2005; Murphy, 2001; Rogers, 2007; Safran, 2002; Spring, 2001; Steinbach, 1997; Stepney, 2001; Wadeson, 2000; White, 2007; Zammit, 2001).

While these books are invaluable for art therapy, the concept of using art according to a specific 'population' is itself problematic because it provides a static definition of clients according to the single parameter of their presenting problem. Additionally all types of problems that define populations are conceptualized differently according to different theories. For example, if addiction is understood as an illness, art will be used to self-regulate the system, but if addiction is understood as a defence against traumatic memories, then art will be used to raise the repressed experience into consciousness. Understanding the type of problem – and thus populations – differs according to the theoretical glasses.

Art therapy books can also be organized according to individual, group, or community settings (Allen, 1995; Betinsky, 1995; Case and Daley, 1990; Docktor, 1994; Henley, 2003; Jones, 2005; Moon, 2002; 2008; Rappaport, 2008; Rogers, 1993; Rubin, 2001; Wadeson, 2000). However, this is also problematic because, as shown in the first section, all theories can be used in all settings; therefore settings are not prescriptive of a single type of art intervention.

Another division of art therapy books is that of general teaching; however, these do not always break down the theory or examples into a set of transparent assumptions about art use (Allen, 1995; Ball, 2002; Betinsky, 1995; Campbell, 1999a; Hogan and Coulter, 2014; Horowitz and Epstein, 2009; Malchiodi, 2007; Moon, 2003; Rubin, 1999; Wadeson, 2000).

Not all of the above divisions define the theoretical assumptions behind the art activities suggested. This creates a danger that the question they answer becomes, 'What should I do with the art?' rather than the question, 'How do I address the problem – and the solution I have identified according to the theoretical glasses that I have committed to – through the art?'

In sum, the claim of this book is that a good understanding of the array of theoretical assumptions in different therapeutic standpoints will, in fact, enable much more choice and richness in art practice than by adhering to a few familiar art activities or general assumptions. These assumptions could be defined as 'absolute truth': for example, that art expresses the unconscious, or that art is relaxing, or that art is good for one, without understanding the theory from which this idea emerged, or its implications for all parts of the therapy. Often, in the public sector, where therapists and clients do not choose but are allocated to one another, the theoretical orientation of the art therapist is not elucidated to the client. The claim of this book is that theory needs to be elucidated and intensified within art therapy training and practice. A clear theoretical base ensures that the 'doing' of art in art therapy emerges coherently from theory, and synchronizes the role of the therapist with the problem and with the solution.

At the same time, in order to create a 'tool box' of theoretical orientations, it is important to reduce the absolute power of the most popular theory because, as stated above, no theory is absolute truth, but rather is a historical and social construct based in a particular location and moment in history. Therapeutic theories in this book are defined as a type of symbolic creation – just like religion, politics, and art, to name a few areas of social creation. All types of therapy aim to help deal with problems in the context of a set of cultural norms and socio-cultural realities. This context and historical moment are paradoxically what created the problem, but also the context within which the solution must be found. In other words, similar to art, cultural and religious theories of therapy is a hermeneutic, creative, and evolving construct that aims to 'heal' or to balance the individual within a given social reality. This includes scientific, humanistic, and social constructs that help people process and react to the complex shifting and often painful realities of their society at a specific time. In terms of art, they are an expression of and also a reaction to a socio-geographic and cultural reality; they aim to both strengthen, but also to balance, or counteract this reality in order to enable the adjustment of the system to a constantly evolving reality. This understanding demystifies theory and enables the therapist to choose the right theory for the social context, population setting, and therapist, and to shift between theories and even use them simultaneously within the same intervention when needed – assuming they are clearly understood at the start.

To exemplify: most problems can be understood through exploring early childhood conflicts and through defence mechanisms used against pain. This takes art as a path to the unconscious, and as an expression of such defence mechanisms (dynamic) most problems can be understood in terms of a person's potential for self-actualization and ability to create meaning out of one's life, using art as a pathway not to the unconscious but to the evolving authentic self (humanistic). Most problems can be analysed in terms of faulty cognitions and ensuing lack of self-regulation, understanding art as a way to envisage solutions and to self-regulate the mind-body connection (CBT and positive psychology). Most problems can also be understood through the roles the clients take within their social systems – understanding art as a space to explore, communicate, and symbolically change these roles and divisions of space (systemic). Most problems are the result of a lack of power and resources within the social world. Thus, from this stance, art helps these sufferers visualize their lack of power and social marginalization, becoming instead the power holders (empowerment and social change). Most problems include an element of conflict and negotiation, where art becomes a distanced transitional space within which to explore conflict.

As an example, let us take the story of Joseph's coat of many colours (Huss, 2009b). Joseph is one of 12 brothers, 10 of whom are his half-brothers born to four different mothers. Joseph's own mother, Rachel, died giving birth to a younger brother. Joseph was his father's favourite son and, consequently, his brothers' most-hated sibling, who threw him into a pit. Joseph's most treasured possession was a coloured coat, a gift from his father, which he wore at all times [Genesis, 37:3]. How can art work with this object, the coat of many colours, through different theories? From a dynamic perspective, the coloured coat could be understood as a transitional object – or in object relations terms, as a metaphor for Joseph's narcissistic compensation for lack of a mother object. From a Jungian perspective, the coat is a kind of mandala, or expression of self; and the pit into which his brothers threw him, can be understood as his meeting with his 'shadow'. From a humanistic perspective, the coat is a metaphor for a young man trying to define his specific 'colours' and holding on to his holistic potential. From a narrative perspective, the coat is a symbol that gives him strength to continue in face of his brothers' rejection. From a CBT perspective, it is a visualization that enables him to hold on to a vision of a brighter future. From a systemic perspective, the coat is an expression of a role within the family system. From a socio-cultural perspective, the coat is an accepted sign of bestowing the social role of leader of the family on to the most suitable child, in the face of competition over who will lead the family; the embroidery shows specific roles according to shape and colour, as in a uniform; and the coat is a cultural way of visually signifying social responsibility to others as well as dominance – as, indeed, Joseph does in the end save the family.

Each of these understandings of Joseph's coat signifies a different meaning for the visual symbol of the colourful coat and may be developed within further art work within the therapy (such as modulating the grandiose brightness of the coat, exploring the meanings of each colour within the coat, or creating coats for others in the family). No single understanding of the colourful coat is the 'truth', and neither is total lack of understanding the truth; rather, each theory may have a moment in the therapy when it becomes most relevant. For example, the moment that the brothers decide to throw him in the pit, or the advent of famine that leads the family to Egypt, clearly demands systemic and social intervention, rather than a dynamic exploration of the past. It may therefore be better to explore his inner world during the times when Joseph is in the pit or in an Egyptian prison. If he is sold into slavery, perhaps a social intervention is what is needed to enable powerholders to release him. If he is wandering around a little lost in his colourful coat, maybe a dynamic or humanistic theory can be used. Often, theories are combined by starting to work on childhood, then to integrate a family approach, to continue to work on negative cognitions as well as on resiliences and to integrate social understandings of the problem. The usefulness of art for the expression of an integrative therapeutic stance is that they can all be anchored within the same art work (Huss *et al.*, 2012a).

Each of the above theories is created within a specific social historical and cultural reality and is constantly evolving within that reality. For example, Freud's libidinal energy theories can be understood as influenced by the industrial revolution that illustrated the theories of repressed energy (Gerken, 2001; Schultz and Schultz, 2011). Similarly, the secularization of society and the rise of science and rational thought versus religion intensified the need to resolve moral and social conflicts internally – between the id (self) and the superego (society) rather than relying on an external religious locus of control, as in the past (Gay, 1989; Leary, 1994).

Within the humanistic theory that followed the dynamic theory after the two world wars, focus on the individual subjective self became relevant in the context of the lack of faith in collective systems, such as the state, and in objective systems, such as 'science'. Art became process-oriented, and individualized creativity was a highly valued activity in education. Similarly, the current shift to short-term and measurable therapy corresponds to the needs of the neo-capitalist market to prove financially viable quick positive outcomes. Developments in science define art as a type of neurological rather than hermeneutic activity and aim to measure its impact on the body.

The above examples are, of course, stereotypical generalizations, but their aim is to demonstrate how theories of therapy and art are created within specific financial and social contexts – and as such are not absolute truths, but ways that people aim to deal with the present reality. Similarly, the concept of beauty in art is constantly evolving, from harmony to interest, to challenge, to cognition, etc., according to the role that art plays in society at a given time and place (Hills, 2001). Art can be understood as a universal act with deep universal 'archetypes' or common denominators of humanity. Alternatively, it is an expression of cultural norms; or, art is a way to fight cultural norms. Additionally, it may be understood as a discrete aesthetic language disconnected from social issues (Rose, 2011). Art can be located within religion (with a spiritual component), within ethnicity, within education, within therapy, or within culture. It can be an expression of the reality of different groups, ranging from the elitist to marginalized sectors of society (Huss, 2009b, 2011, 2012a, 2012b). These 'cultural versus universal' or 'crafts versus art' or 'process versus product' dichotomies can be broken down into varying roles of art emerging from the theory within which it is used. From this, therefore, art can have many different roles within art therapy.

In sum, the first point made above, was the importance of theories; the second, was that while theories are so important, it is also necessary to understand them not as an absolute reality, but as a creative type of problem solving within a specific context. The third point is that in accordance with the first two theories, each theory is also a constantly evolving interpretation of itself and understands the role of art differently within therapy. From this, art therapists can utilize different uses of art according to different theories, rather than according to different activities, materials, or populations.

Organization of the book

The first section of the book will first outline a set of theories in detail, including: dynamic, Jung, object relations, ego psychology, humanistic, gestalt, narrative, mind-body CBT, systemic, empowerment, and social change theories. These roughly divide into dynamic, humanistic, and social-systemic theories. Each of these three general categories will have its own summary, showing how the conceptions and uses of art and of the therapist shift within the theoretical epistemology. These are not inclusive of all theories used in art therapy, but rather aim to show how to translate a theory into practical art therapy.

Each chapter will have the following components:

- contribution of the theory to art therapy
- the theory
- problems as defined by the theory
- the solutions as defined by the theory
- the social context
- macro applications
- role of art in this theory
- dynamic art therapy
- role of the art therapist
- evaluation
- art evaluation
- supervision
- research
- critique of the theory
- central concepts exemplified through case study
- working the theory: art therapy skills and techniques
- verbal techniques
- visual techniques: art setting, process, and interpretation
- overall skills to practise
- art-based skills to practise.

It is important to state here that these are this author's interpretations of the theory and are not presumed to be the only single way to interpret the theory, or to encompass all that has been written about art therapy from each perspective, or to include all of the theories outlined in art therapy. The art therapy literature in each field is extensive, constantly growing and evolving even while writing this book. Thus, the art therapy literature in this book is by no means the most encompassing or the most important literature, but rather is used to exemplify the integrative theoretical standpoint outlined in this book.

Each chapter will be illustrated using a case study of a group of women who experienced sexual abuse in childhood. The reason for using the same case study is to demonstrate how the same art work can be understood through different theories. The case study will be introduced before the theories, and will be summarized at the end of the introduction.

The second section of the book aims to model how to think of specific issues or areas in art therapy, through different theoretical lenses. The various areas include:

Chapter 14   Art setting and materials, processes, and interpretation.
Chapter 15   Settings, from micro to macro, that is, working with individuals, families, groups, and communities.
Chapter 16   Working with different populations, including inherent problems, (such as physical mental and emotional disabilities) and environmental problems (such as trauma, abuse, and transitions).
Chapter 17   Evaluation, supervision and research of art therapy.

Readers may either delve into a specific theory in the first section or use an overview of the issue that most concerns them. The aim of the second section is to model how considerations of working with a specific population, setting, material, or supervision can be conceptualized dynamically through different theories, rather than statically. For example, working with an autistic client can be conceptualized statically as a population A – that demands intervention B – or can be conceptualized in many ways according to different theories. The aim is thus to demonstrate how to choose and shift between theories, and how to utilize them to enlarge understanding and choice within specific art therapy settings, populations, and interactions. The systematic analysis of discrete elements of art therapy such as population, through different theories, raises interesting questions about basic assumptions of art therapy that are discussed in these chapters.

Introduction to the case study

In the first section of the book, the central concepts of each theory will be exemplified with images from the following case study of an art therapy group of sexually abused women.

The case study of these women has been outlined in further detail in a previous publication (Huss, 2010). The aim here is to illustrate central concepts in all of the theories, demonstrating how the same images can be analysed through each.

The women in the case study signed consent forms to have their art work presented under false names and with no identifying features. The original research using these images underwent the university ethics committee.

The following is an outline of each of the four women whose images are presented

A) *Shoshana* was sexually abused as a child over a few years by a relative. Furthermore, as a religious girl, it was expected in her culture that she should become pregnant immediately after her marriage, but when this failed Shoshana learnt that she and her husband were in need of special medical treatment to assist them. She experienced the gyneacological treatments as an additional 'invasion of her body'. Shoshana was ambivalent about pregnancy in general, although she very much wanted children. This ambivalence was not culturally acceptable and she could not talk about it with her family or husband. She decided over the year of being with the art therapy group, that she would put off having a baby until she felt more comfortable about it.

Over time, her images became more flexible and colourful and the black centre that she called 'the blackness', identified as her sexual abuse and womb, was replaced by an image of the baby that she wanted. After a year she decided to start medical treatment to become pregnant.

Figure A1 was her first image, and she called it 'blackness'. *'I don't have words to describe my image, I can only draw blackness.'*

Figure A2 was her second image, showing squares with a 'black' centre that she defined as 'the blackness'. Shoshana added the words of a popular song about how unjust the world is on top of the coloured squares.

Figure A1   Shoshana's drawings

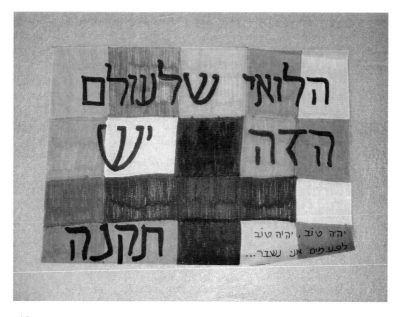

Figure A2

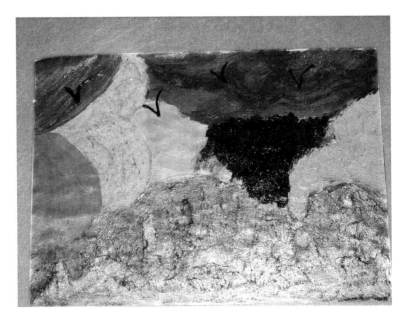

Figure A3

Figure A3 is another image with a black centre. Shohsana stated that the colours have become a view of hills that she loves and that give her comfort.

Figure A4 was drawn towards the end of the group and includes coloured squares around the centre with a baby, instead of a black shape. This was when Shoshana decided to start fertility treatment.

B) *Rina* is a Russian immigrant who was sexually abused by a relative when she was young. The relative continued to live at home and Rina would present either a 'tough' tomboy facade, or an exaggeratedly female stance. Within the group she often told stories of situations of intense danger with men that she encountered, but was emotionally disconnected from these stories. The present concerns that she raised in the group included her uncertainty about staying in her job as a security guard. Rina's images were often split into black and white, or half images (see figures B1 and B2). Over time her pictures became more integrated and softer, and she left her 'tough' job and her 'tough' boyfriend.

Figure B1 is an image divided by black and colour. '*This is life – black or a sunny beach.*'

Figure B2 is an image of a woman without a face, also split in half. '*I feel like this woman sometimes, split into two.*'

Figure B3 is a doodle incorporating shadows and light. '*Here I just let myself draw, a doodle, but it has a blacker area and a lighter area, although it's more integrated.*'

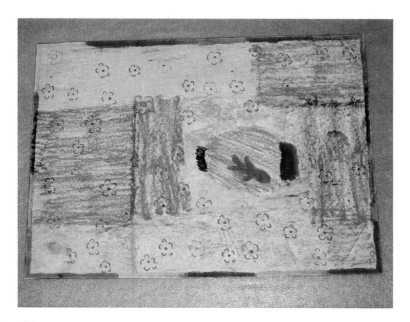

Figure A4

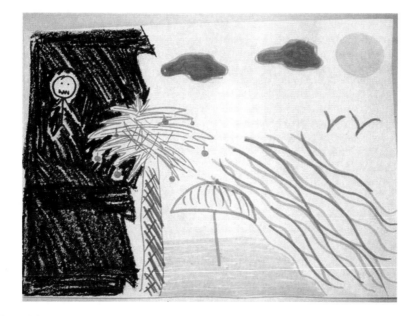

Figure B1 Rina's drawings

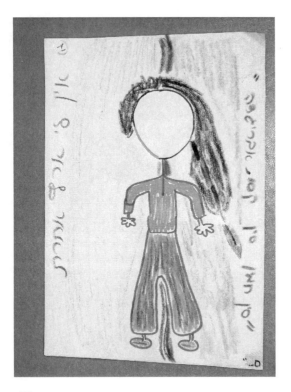

Figure B2

Figure B4 is a mandala of merging black and colour. *'Here, the black and colour are together, – that's how I want it to be.'*

C) *Sharon* is a very beautiful young girl, who was abused by a neighbour who looked after her as a child. She always smiled and behaved, in the group's words, like a 'Barbie doll'. In time she stated that she felt 'like ice inside'. At the beginning, Sharon drew repetitive disconnected shapes and filled in different empty spaces. She gradually added a little girl into one of the images that was much discussed in the group.

Figure C1 is a repeated shape of boxes that are half open on a background of dots. Sharon stated that she felt calm by drawing this doodle.

Figure C2 is a doodle that has a circular shape emerging from the centre. Sharon stated that she enjoyed drawing this circular doodle.

Figure C3 is an image of a girl, also surrounded by dots and outreached hands, with a red spot on her skirt.

When asked, she stated that the hands reaching out the girl were trying to help her.

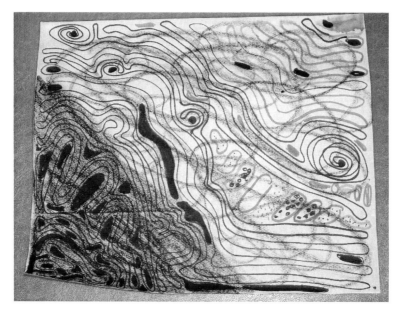

Figure B3

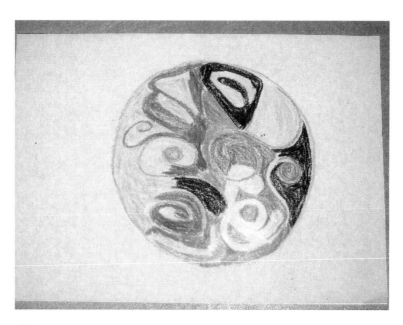

Figure B4

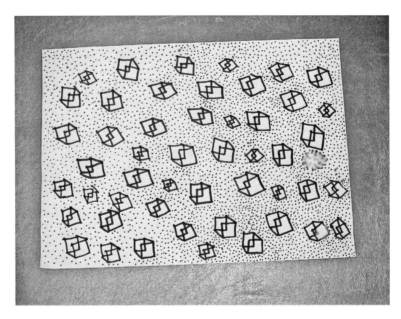

Figure C1 Sharon's drawings

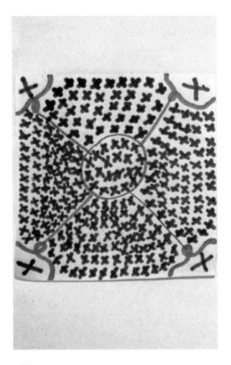

Figure C2

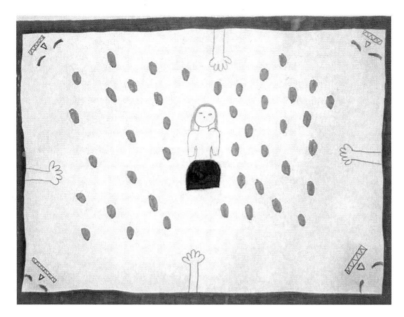

Figure C3

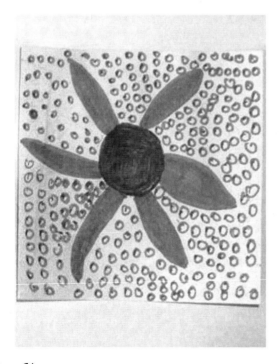

Figure C4

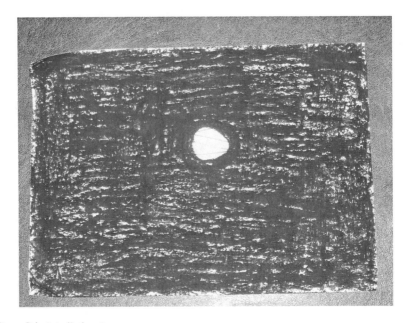

Figure D1 Avital's drawings

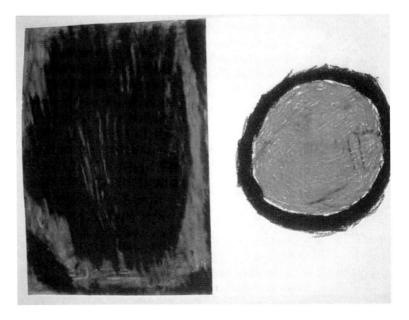

Figure D2

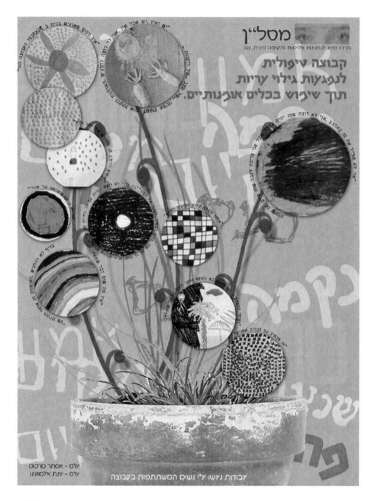

Figure D3

Another woman in the group confronted her, pointing out that 'The hands are not helping, they could also be understood as attacking ... the hands are attacking and no one is help-ing – also the girl is hurt.'

Figure C4 is an additional doodle of coloured circular shapes but also with a flower in the middle. Sharon stated that she enjoyed creating the images and seeing how they were developing.

D) *Avital* is a woman in her 50s, older than the others, and married with children. She was abused by her father as a child. Her father had died and she only recently started remembering the abuse. She is a strong mother figure, looking after her five children and the others in the group, along with her old sick mother. Although she gave advice and nurturing to others, at first Avital refused to draw at all – just as she refused to take up 'space' in the group – saying that she had no idea how to draw. Eventually she represented herself by leaving a small white dot on a tiny piece of paper covered in black (Figure D1). She exclaimed '*There, that's me, I don't exist.*'

Over time, as stated above, she experienced more anger, and depicted it with the colour red (Figure D2). She later defined her anger and also her energy as her decision to become a social activist.

Eventually, at the end of the year, with the help of the rape crisis centre, she made a poster incorporating all of the women's images shown above (and others) (Figure D3). The poster was used as advocacy for the centre, and Avital ran a session of lectures using it to raise awareness of sexual abuse in different welfare communities and educational frames, and to try to advocate more serious punishment for perpetrators. Avital stated that she wanted to teach women about the experience.

Section 1

Art therapy according to theory

A

ART AS DECODING THE UNCONSCIOUS: INTRODUCTION TO ART THERAPY THROUGH DYNAMIC THEORY

The dynamic meta-theories define problems and solutions as being based within inner conflicts between id, ego, and superego, and as entrenched within the defences used against these conflicts, which become calcified within early childhood. The solution becomes to reach awareness and understanding of these suppressed conflicts, by raising them to consciousness. Humanity is thus, on the one hand, riddled with inner conflicts, but on the other, is able to apply its conscious mind to interpret and to solve them. Art in the dynamic theory, broadly defined as the use of metaphor, symbols, visions, dreams, and sensual information, will be shown to have the vital role of making the unconscious, conscious. In object relations, art makes the relationship visible and creates a symbolic zone within which to enact it. Winnicott (1958, 1991) connected the content and relationship as interacting within the symbolic spaces, tightening the triangle of art therapy – therapist, client and art. Art is the vital transitional symbolic space within which people can individuate and connect to others, and within which relationships are worked through. Using ego psychology, art's role is further developed into the proactive role of being able to negotiate between id and superego, and to enable adaptive defences such as sublimation instead of dissociation.

Jung's theories of culturally located archetypes also enable art to heal intrinsically, outside the zone of therapy, as part of the symbolic resources of a culture. Thus, art shifts from an expression of pathology in the self or in relationships in Freud's theory and in object relations, to a way to negotiate and to integrate conflicts in ego psychology and in Jungian theories. This in effect illustrates the shift from art psychotherapy to art as therapy, showing that the various dynamic interpretations of the basic theory provide a varied and flexible range for using art. Each sub-theory or interpretation of Freudian theory has evolved in relation to shifting social realities of modernism, the grand theories, a belief in the rational versus religious mind, in science, industry, the emergence of childhood as a discrete concept, the struggle of women to leave the home and enter the workforce, colonialism, and the changing roles of art after the invention of the camera, among others. These chapters will show how Freudian and object relations theories focus on the relationship, while ego psychology and Jungian theories focus on the art.

From the perspective of the rigid humanistic meta-theories, in which this theory can be critiqued, the client is unable to be the interpreter of his own art. From a mind-body and CBT orientation, the dynamic theory is based on myths

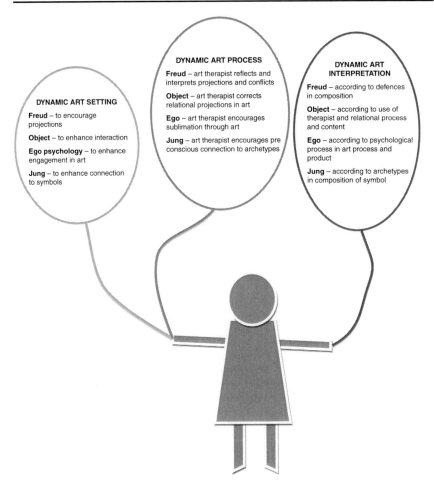

DYNAMIC ART SETTING

Freud – to encourage projections

Object – to enhance interaction

Ego psychology – to enhance engagement in art

Jung – to enhance connection to symbols

DYNAMIC ART PROCESS

Freud – art therapist reflects and interprets projections and conflicts

Object – art therapist corrects relational projections in art

Ego – art therapist encourages sublimation through art

Jung – art therapist encourages pre conscious connection to archetypes

DYNAMIC ART INTERPRETATION

Freud – according to defences in composition

Object – according to use of therapist and relational process and content

Ego – according to psychological process in art process and product

Jung – according to archetypes in composition of symbol

Figure 1.1 Dynamic theories: setting, process, and interpretation

and narratives that do not exist and thus cannot be proven, and does not focus on clients' strengths and cognitions. From a critical social perspective, the universalistic standpoint of the theory discounts cultural constructions of reality and of art. However, if these theories are understood as a creation of a specific time and place within history, then their huge contribution to art therapy can be continued. This includes the centrality of creativity as a path to resolve problems and to reach inner experience, the creative, intuitive, and hermeneutic focuses of the therapist and client within therapy, the meanings attributed to symbols, metaphors, and elusive projective processes. According to dynamic theory, art is a central means to address and to express pain, desire, and love, which situates art therapy within its natural home in the world of fine art, humanities, and visual culture – even if Freud took such pains to define art as science. Figure 1.1 outlines the variations within this theory that will be explored within this section.

Chapter 1

Art as a path to the unconscious
Art therapy and psychodynamic therapy

The contribution of the dynamic theory is the central role it plays within art therapy; it creates a rich tapestry of therapeutic interaction, including non-linear content, and the conceptualization of the relationship, form, and content as parallel and interactive zones of intervention. According to this theory, the process of therapy itself is creative, intuitive, and process-oriented. Art is given a vital role within the developing psyche.

According to the dynamic theory, humanity deals with deep inner conflicts created by sexual and primal drives, which are in opposition to the socializing demands of society. People are primal energy, and society is the 'machine' that represses this energy. People have to navigate between their primal drives (the 'id'), and their conscience (the 'superego') with the help of the ego – which is caught between them. These inner conflicts are so painful that strong defences are created to cope with them in childhood. The defences become calcified and hinder the ability to work through emotions. However, these basic libidinal energies may also be sublimated and used in productive ways when more flexible defences are adopted. The place where inner conflicts become calcified is in the early socialization of children, as they pass through the oral, anal, and oedipal stages of development. Each stage demands a dramatic negotiation between desire and culture, in terms of level of self-regulation of oral and anal drives, denunciation of omnipotence, sexual desires, jealousy, and conquests. Unresolved conflicts from these stages become introjected and are projected on to adult relationships (Fontana, 1993; Freud, 1900, 1936, 1997; Gay, 1989).

Problems may be defined as the conflict between id and superego, as well as the defences used against these conflicts. The defences against pain are themselves often the symptoms, or presenting problem.

The solution is in people's ability, while riddled with inner conflicts, to apply their rational mind to these conflicts to overcome them by understanding them. These inner unconscious conflicts and defences are raised to consciousness with the help of the therapist, and are understood, thus diminishing the conflict and making its defence unnecessary (Berry, 2000; Freud, 1900; Gay, 1989; Higdon, 2004).

The social context in which dynamic theories were conceived was that of a traditional society in transition to a secular society, and shifts from religious to scientific epistemologies. Thus, there was a loss of religion as an external organizing locus of control, and humanity had to control its own drives from within, with the help of the ego. The advances in science, and the industrial revolution it created, searched for a 'science' of the mind. Metaphors of repressed and then released energy in industry can be understood as a concept transferred to the human psyche through the id as pure energy, the ego as the breaks, and superego as pushing down the energy similar to a machine. The modernist notion of science, consciousness and understanding as enabling control over the world and the self, and as the foundation for the resolution of unconscious conflicts, were at the base of this conception. The therapist, therefore, as a 'blank' invisible screen but able to interpret everything from an invisible omnipotent standpoint, becomes a type of godlike figure (Kvale, 1992; Leary, 1994).

Macro applications of Freud's theory of defences, projections, and regressions may be applied to whole communities as well as to individuals. For example, racism towards groups may be understood as a defence of displacement of unwanted parts of the self onto the 'other' (Said, 1978); or relations with a leader may hold elements of projections or splits onto parents. Societies can sublimate aggression into art and culture, or express it directly through war (Mitchell, 1995).

The role of art in this theory to access the elusive unconscious is, according to Freud's topological theory, defined as a central method, together with dreams, jokes, and slips of the tongue. Artistic activity is thus fed by the id, and is a regressive projection of hidden desires, but it is also an important intuitive place that can access the inner self. Artists are, on the one hand, seen as lacking in superego, unable to effectively repress primary drives; and on the other, they can be understood as having a unique intuitive ability to connect to the unconscious and to express it (Freud, 1936; Leary, 1994).

The connection between art and emotional or psychological states was not only strengthened by Freud, but also by then-current developments in the art world (Rubin, 1999). This includes the invention of the camera, which helped to push art into an expressive and emotional, rather than documenting role (Hills, 2001). Furthermore, art was used as a way to occupy the abundance of wounded and traumatized patients in psychiatric hospitals after the two world wars, and its therapeutic value was conceptualized together with the Freudian understanding of art (Rubin, 1999; Waller, 1993).

Dynamic art therapy is based on the central concept of projection in dynamic theory into art therapy, with the therapist working in three simultaneous projective zones: those of the relationship, the therapy setting, and the art activity (Schaverien, 1999). Within the art work, the process, product, and reaction to the product are all additional projective zones; therefore the art intensifies the projective and regressive potential of the therapy (Case and Daley, 1990; Kramer, 1971; Naumberg, 1966). Art therapists aim to utilize art to reach unconscious content. This can be in relation to process, product, reaction to product, and projections on to the therapist in relation to art making. Art is thus considered a potentially regressive activity that encourages connection to early conflicts.

According to this theory the role of the art therapist is to encourage the expression of, and then to interpret inner childhood conflicts, desires, defence mechanisms, and projections, as they are expressed in the content of the art and the therapy relationship, and in present problems. The therapist aims to maintain a neutral persona that enables the client to project his early conflicted relationships in a transference process. The therapist achieves this by analysing their own reactions to the client, or counter-transferable projections back onto the client, with the help of supervision, in order to create a neutral screen. The art is another place where the projected relationship is expressed (Waller, 1993). The projective triangle of art, client, and therapist is activated as different interactive symbolic zones within which to express conflicts, defences, and projections.

If, according to dynamic theory, evaluation is based on the inner conflicts and defences in light of early childhood experiences, then the gradual unravelling of these elements into the consciousness of the client may be evaluated over time in terms of the client's developing the ability to accept interpretations of these desires and conflicts and understand their relationship to early childhood unresolved conflicts – and the ensuing disappearance of symptoms. Evaluation is the responsibility of the therapist, rather than the client. For example, even if the client states that the therapy is not working or symptoms are becoming worse, the therapist may understand this as part of the process that includes defence against new content, and not a reason to stop the therapy. The client's progress can be evaluated according to their ability to accept the therapist's interpretations, according to the reduction of symptoms as well as to increased insight.

Projective art tests are a central art-based evaluative method, based on the assumption that the unconscious content will emerge with the compositional elements of the images. This includes the use of abstract projective shapes, and also more structured projective techniques, such as house–tree–people drawings; elements all considered to be projections of self (Burns, 1987; Silver, 2005; Wilson, 2001).

The concept behind art evaluation tests is that clients cannot self-report on unconscious elements of their personality or on defence mechanisms used, but these will be manifest within the compositional elements of their drawings. Thus, if asked to draw basic images such as a house, a tree or a person, they will project unconscious desires and conflicts, as well as defences, onto the composition of these elements. Purely compositional evaluations address elements such as overall size, location, and line and shading quality. For example, a too small drawing of a person expresses depression, while a too large drawing expresses narcissistic compensation. These may all be analysed as stress, or, as an expressions of defences against the stress.

For instance, butterflies and other positive elements in a drawing can express distraction from a problem; drawing a person of the opposite sex symbolizes sexual concerns; large eyes, paranoia; and poor compositional integration impulsivity; shading, anxiety (e.g. large mouth and buttons, as oral fixation). A focus of composition on the upper right-hand side expresses optimism, while a focus on the lower right-hand side expresses depression (content elements include bizarre placedment versus realism in form and colour, etc). Determinates of mood are analysed according to assumption that depression and withdrawal will use dark colours, or lack of colour, while impulsive and uncontrolled natures will use strong colours (Burns, 1987; Burns and Kaufman, 1972; Brooke, 1996; Cohen, 1994; Feder and Feder, 1999; Furth, 1998; Silver, 2005; Wilson, 2001).

However, there is much controversy concerning the reliability of projective drawing tests overall because they have been found to be problematic in terms of validity. For example, more pathology was found in lower-class people when using the research, and the types of training of the psychologist determined similarity in evaluation (Handler and Thomas, 2003; Kapitan, 2003). They are usually used as part of an overall and tentative evaluation of a client using clinical judgement, after which they can help the psychologist to shift to compositional elements.

Supervision is central and parallel to the therapy in that it enables a 'blank screen' for the therapist to understand and unravel the multiple levels of projection – on to both the art and the therapist. This can include using some of the therapist's art work to understand unconscious elements in the therapy relationship and in the parallel process between therapist and supervisor. It will conceive of the supervising space as parallel to the therapy, in terms of being a safe emotional container for the therapist, as well as a place to explore the therapist's projections on to the client, and on to the client's art work. The supervisor will invest in creating a relationship of trust, and activating an interpretation of symbolic content that emerges in order to understand the central problem.

Research is based on analysing therapeutic interactions according to the dynamic meta-theory. This can include descriptive and hermeneutic case studies, where the therapist interprets the client's art-making activity and products as well as the projective relationship between them. This correlates to the power of the therapist to analyse his client within the practice.

One critique of the dynamic meta-theory is that, overall, it is rigid and does not enable the client to be the interpreter of his own art. Another problem is that it is based on unsubstantiated myths and narratives. There is no 'unconscious' in the physical body. However, many art therapy programmes are based on this theory as an absolute or single truth, or as a way to analyse art, rather than as a specific prism to understand art. Another problem is that the universalistic stance of the theory discounts cultural constructions of reality, as well as marginalizing women's intelligence and sexuality (Berry, 2000; Freud, 1900; Gay, 1989; Higdon, 2004; Kvale, 1992; Leary, 1994).

Its pessimistic focus on childhood conflicts as being calcified and thus deterministic is also a problematic concept. The concept of consciousness or insight as being sufficient to solve a problem is questionable when thinking of temperamental and neurological problems. For example, for many years autism was understood dynamically as the result of an over-controlling mother. This type of therapy enables self-development, but demands long-term and expensive therapy that makes it exclusive to middle-class clients. The focus on problems as disconnected from society is also problematic from a social lens (Todd, 2007).

Central concepts exemplified through case study

Reflection and interpretation

Dynamic theories employ very delicate modes of intervention, such as active listening and reflection, and also very intense modes of intervention, such as interpretation according to the dynamic meta-theory.

> Sharon (3A) repeatedly drew boxes that were half open. The art therapist reflected that her motions when drawing were repetitive and seemed to take her away emotionally from the group, although they calmed her as a form of dissociation.
>
> The art therapist interpreted the final image as boxes that didn't have a base and so they could not hold anything. This reflects her wish to be contained, and protected by her mother (and by the group) that she feels cannot be fulfilled, and so the boxes are open.

Transference and counter-transference

These are projections and counter-projections of the client onto the therapist and therapist onto the client. These can be expressed in all elements of the therapy, including body language, words, behaviour, art processes, art products, and reactions to the art of both client and therapist. The inclusion of art enables an additional zone to project onto, and an additional distanced zone within which to react to these projections.

> The therapist experienced a feeling of fear when she looked at Rina's (3C) image of hands reaching out to 'help' (but in fact to abuse) the girl in the centre of the image. The therapist realized that this anxiety was a projection of what the young girl-Rina in the image had felt. Rina stated that the hands were 'helping' – a reaction formation that denied the experience of hands abusing her – and this inner fear was projected on to the therapist and experienced by her.

Regression

Art processes enable regression to early stages of development that in turn enable access to early calcified conflicts.

> Avital (D2) scribbled intensely with the red and black oil pastels, expressing anger and regressing to an earlier developmental stage in terms of her art work. She expressed her repressed anger at her sexual abuse through making a 'mess'.

Defences

Defences are the ways in which we try to deny painful feelings such as loss, shame, and guilt. As small children, our defences can be simple and rigid, while as we grow up and reach insight, we can move to more sophisticated and adaptive defences.

For example, dissociation or somatization can be extreme defences that cut one off totally from the painful experience, and thus from parts of the self and from reality. Conversely, denial, reaction formation, or rationalization can be more adaptive. Sublimation and integration are defences that transform the primary pain.

> *At the beginning, all of the examples in the case study (ABCD) show intense defences in the art, such as types of boundaries (elements not touching each other on the page); levels of control (intense neatness and using only felt-tip pens that enable full control). These are defences that express efforts to distract from anxiety (filling in the page, repetitions). The images became a place to raise these defences to consciousness, and to confront them. Over time, all art works became more flexible, with shapes touching and colours connected, showing a move to more adaptive defences.*

Art as an expression of both unconscious content and defences

Art expression can be understood as a 'crack' in defences but also as an expression of defences, as shown in Rima's example of the 'helping' hands.

> *In Rima's image of dots with a girl in the middle (3C), the dots express the defence mechanism of dissociation as repetition of shapes that is calming. However, the red dot on the girl's skirt can be interpreted as an expression of the sexual abuse that 'slipped' out of the defences. This red dot became a visual confrontation with the defence.*

Working the theory: art therapy skills and techniques

Verbal techniques

A central technique is active listening – which demands full attention to recurring words, metaphors, and themes; and active looking in terms of recurring symbols, compositional elements, or reactions to the art work. These are returned to the client through reflection, that is, the ability to contemplate the client's content, without adding any interpretation, feedback, or advice. This might include repeating the content; paraphrasing and summarizing it; focusing on emotional or cognitive content; reflecting on it; and asking open questions. Questions may be to ask for clarification or to expand metaphors, symbols in the language or in the art work. Alternatively the reflection may constitute being silent but actively listening and observing. Within this silence, the therapist needs to work on the constant processing of emotional reactions to the client and to the art work and on the interpretation of projections and content of both verbal and visual elements.

Thus, although the therapist may not be saying a lot, he or she is actively processing the client's and his or her own reactions. In contrast with the above described 'quiet' but effective forms of reflection, the dynamic art therapist can choose times to use interpretation of the content, composition, and reaction of the client to the art work.

Another area of interpretation is that of gaps between different elements (such as content and composition, or verbal versus visual content). This includes pointing out the defence mechanisms, and the stuck childhood conflicts as expressed in art making, product, and interpretation and reaction to therapist. Connecting these conflicts to present ones is a further means of interpretation. On this level, the therapist can be defined as creative, using a 'third ear' to notice recurring metaphors, slips, and non-linear connections between elements in the words and in the images. This provides multiple zones of interpretation to work with (Huss and Cwikel, 2008a; Naumberg, 1966; Rose, 2011).

Visual techniques

Setting

In order to encourage projection, the setting and the art, just like the therapist, will aim to be neutral, with a free choice of basic art materials (e.g. clay and paint rather than cuttings from magazines and stickers). The level of fluidity or controllability of materials that the client chooses, their associations as parts of the body, or their inherent characteristics, will be understood as part of the projection of the client on to the material. The art use will be non-directive, to enable free projection on to art materials and processes (such as choosing a very fluid childlike art material – or only pencils). Primary and regressive materials, a suitable room, and tolerance of mess, will enable regressive processes that show childhood conflicts that have become calcified (Case and Daley 1990; Dalley *et al.*, 1993; Kramer, 1971; Landgarten, 2013; Naumberg, 1966).

Process

As stated, the art use will be non-directive to enable free projection on to art materials and processes; and process, product and reaction to product will be constantly reflected and interpreted by the art therapist's observation but not intervention. Regression through art materials, to access these experiences, will be encouraged. The art therapist will reflect and interpret these processes (Case and Daley 1990; Dalley *et al.*, 1993; Kramer, 1971; Landgarten, 2013; Naumberg 1966).

Interpretation of art products

The client's use of the therapist while making art will be understood as internalized relationship desires (e.g. yearning for a mother figure by being helpless in relation to the art directives; or excessive independence as lack of trust; or competitiveness with art therapist as oedipal fixation; or use of too much paint as oral fixation; or attention to clearing up as anal fixation). The interpretation according to the aforementioned psychodynamic meta-theory is applied to all components of therapy, including verbal and real-life interactions (e.g. what is the meaning of the client being late) the art process (why the materials are 'never enough') the art products (why the adult has long pointed hands) and the interpretations (why the client constantly belittles his own art work). This creates a multiple interpretive zone. Thus, the therapist, the room, the art process, product, and reactions to the art process are all symbolic zones for interpretation of defences, conflicts, and childhood fixations. This in effect creates a type of 'hall of mirrors' where everything is bounced back from everything. A central analytical focus for art therapists can be the discrepancies between these different zones. This is the dynamic 'triangle' of art therapy, where the zones of transference, projection, and interpretation can occur between the client and therapist, between the client and art work, or between the therapist and art work, and each can express different things. This interpretive process is constantly fed back to the client and thus interpretation is an ongoing activity of the therapist within the art-making process.

Overall skills to practise

Working with self and with counter-transference: Dynamic therapists need to undergo dynamic therapy to work with their counter-transferences. They need to understand their personal issues, defences, and calcified childhood stages. It is important to ensure that there is supervision within this theory, as that is the place to understand them. The therapist can use their own art work to access this information.

Learning to accept regression, defensive behaviour, and ambiguity in the process includes the therapist's need to tolerate the client's regressive, resistant, and often difficult projections, as well as the 'stuck' times, and to build a gradual interpretation of what is happening.

Working with symbolic listening: As described above, learning to listen actively and creatively to content, composition, and projections in both words and art work simultaneously demands deep concentration, even though from the outside it may look as if nothing is happening.

Learning to address both content and composition simultaneously within art work: Learn to 'read' the content and symbolic level, and also the compositional level of art works, and shift between them. The diagnostic literature can help gain sensitivity to shading, contours, encapsulations, repetitions, transparencies, barriers, cut of pages, out of context elements, overall organization of the composition, and others. It can also include noticing feelings that the client is creating in the self, and reactions to the client (Furth, 1998; Kramer, 1971; Robbins 1999).

Learning to give interpretations indirectly through additional metaphors: Especially with children, the interpretations can be presented through metaphors and art engagement.

Art-based skills to practise

Projections: Choose someone who arouses strong emotions in you. Create an image of that person. Identify what is being projected onto that person, and create an image of the original person. Note the differences between the real and the current character.

Conflict and childhood: Create an image of a stage of childhood that you think was most difficult for you. Connect it to a present conflict.

Defences as against pain: Create an image of the loss or difficulty that you are experiencing at present, and analyse the gaps between content and composition, and how the composition expresses your defences as against the pain. Then, create an image of your defence as a small animal, and befriend it.

Chapter 2

Art as relationships

Art therapy and object relations

A contribution of object relations to art therapy is the connection between relationships and symbolic spaces, which is central to art therapy in that it bridges art – or symbolic interaction and relational elements – to cognition and emotion, creating a rich base for art therapy theory. With his concept of transitional space, Winnicott focused on how characteristics of the introjected relationship are projected on to symbolic transitional objects and spaces that help the client to engage with, and also to separate from, the real object. Transitional space is the playful zone within which one learns to interact with people, and to internalize positive concepts of self and of other (Winnicott, 1958, 1991). The development of this ability to symbolize relationships encompasses cognitive, emotional, and relational intelligences. In art therapy, it explains the intense triangular connection between therapist, client, and art.

Object relations theory focuses on the relationship between therapist and clients, with their art supporting this relationship. It focuses on the impact of internalizations of important relationships in the client's life that are introjected and re-enacted within present relationships. Through the relationship with the other, the self is created. The concept of a relationship with the mother, according to this theory, is different from that in Freud's theory, which focuses on sexual and oedipal drives; but rather it conceives of the holistic combination of trust, predictability, and love (Ainsworth, 1969; Bowlby, 1990; Coleman and Farris-Dufrene, 1996; Fairbairn, 1954; Fishler *et al.*, 1990; Gomez, 1997; Higdon, 2004; Winnicott, 1958, 1991). More specifically, Melanie Klein focused on internalizations of the mother that include intense splits between aggression and love. This ambivalence has to be resolved by going through a depressive stage to create an integrated gestalt of other – and from that of self (Klein, 1932). Bowlby pointed to the biological importance of imprinting a set person, whose interaction becomes predictable. This constant loving relationship is shown as vital for physical development to occur. On a less drastic level, object constancy enables the development of trust in others, and in the self (Bowlby 1990). Winnicott (1958) developed the idea of the interplay between identification and individuation as occurring in the interaction and slips in interaction with the mother, and thus the ability to separate from the 'good enough mother', who is mostly attuned to her child, but sometimes not. By learning to tolerate frustration and loneliness in small amounts, people reach the ability to connect and to individuate

The problem is the lack of this safe person and safe space within which to build trust in relationships, and from this to individuation and trust in self. The solution is to become aware of the impact of these deficits in early relationships, and to separate them from the present relationships, through focusing on what happens in the projections on to the therapist and in the transitional symbolic zone of the therapy space (Ainsworth, 1969; Bowlby, 1990; Coleman and Farris-Dufrene, 1996; Fairbairn, 1954; Fishler *et al.*, 1990; Gomez, 1997; Higdon, 2004; Winnicott, 1958, 1991).

The social context scrutinizes the mother relationship, which can be analysed from a feministic perspective as a strategy to return women home from the jobs they took over in the wars. Another shift was the rise of the concept of childhood as separate from adulthood, as expressed in compulsory education and children's rights (Kvale, 1992; Leary, 1994; Robinson, 1993).

Macro theories can be conceptualized as the ways in which society creates transitional spaces or symbolic zones for working through collective experiences, and negotiation of connection and individuation. For example, spontaneous collective mourning rituals, such as flowers put on famous people's graves, can be understood as a symbolic space to enable mourning and separation. Indeed, flags can be seen as a type of transitional object signifying national togetherness. Transitional space as a symbolic zone is applied within art-based conflict resolution. Meeting symbolically is a safe and distanced way to humanize the other, and to overcome negative projections and splits. Projections of groups on to leaders, splitting people into good–bad can also be analysed through object relations (Spivak and Guha, 1988; Waller, 1993; Winnicott, 1991).

The role of art in this theory becomes focused on the creative and interactive processes of art making, symbolizing, and exploring meanings and relationships through art, rather than on analysing the art product (Case and Daley, 1990; Dalley *et al.*, 1993; Malchiodi, 1998b; Robbins, 1999; Waller, 1993).

Object relations translate into art therapy through Winnicott's theory (1958) of transitional space that provides a strong role for art and plays as a space within which to actively symbolize and work through primary relationships in order to understand them, gain control over them, and to change them within the symbolic space. The role of art can be understood as a symbolic space in which to act out and to access introjections of primary relationships, as in the dynamic theories already mentioned. For example, if females are always drawn as witch-like, or always as angels, by a client then this can express an unresolved split in the introjection of the mother figure, and art can be used to further explore and integrate these splits. Art becomes a space in which to communicate and also to negotiate similarities and differences between people. The art object (such as the teddy bear) also becomes a symbol of a relationship through intense projections. Winnicott (1958) shows how relationships are held and internalized by giving them symbolic shape and containers; at the same time, symbolic containers or the ability to symbolize are also what enable relationships to form (Winnicott, 1958).

The role of the art therapist is to focus on the relationship transference on to themselves as expressed through interaction around the art, showing attachment styles and introjections of former object relations. For example, by creating a predictable setting and persona, the therapist creates the 'transitional space' within which there is enough trust to deal with painful emotions.

Evaluation includes interpreting relationship issues through a client's behaviour and through art, and evaluating changes in introjected relationships through the relationship projected on to the therapist. Another area of evaluation can be the growing ability to utilize play and creativity to work through relationship issues and ability to tolerate both connection and individuation in art processes and products (Furth, 1998; Robbins, 1999; Rubin, 1999; Winnicott, 1958).

Supervision includes identifying the described relational issues, and working on transference – of client and counter-transference of therapist – as a parallel process in the supervision, as well as thinking of ways to create the transitional spaces and to enhance art work (Higdon, 2004; Robbins, 1999; Rubin, 1999).

Research will be based on hermeneutic case studies that show the holistic use of art and therapist in terms of meta-theories of relational projections and shifts, rather than on diagnosing art in terms of defences and drives, as in the former chapter (Case and Daley, 1995; Dalley *et al.*, 1993; Robbins, 1999; Waller, 1993; Winnicott, 1958)

A critique of this theory, as in general dynamic theory, is that it focuses exclusively on the mother–child relationship, with a deterministic focus on early relationships, rather than assuming that relationships can constantly be corrected over a lifetime, rather than introjected (Hamilton, 1989; Kvale, 1992; Viney and King, 1998).

Central concepts exemplified through case study

Projections

As described in the first chapter, the assumption is that former relationships are projected on to current ones, and also on to the art work and therapist (Freud, 1936).

> *Avital (D) projected her need for mothering on to others, being a caretaker for everyone. She found it hard to accept the art therapist as someone she could lean on and at the beginning often competed with the therapist's role. Over time she began to trust the therapist and this enabled her to start to explore her identity in art.*

Introjected relationships

These are our primary relationships, which are internalized and become part of the self. For example, if a parent is very critical, then one develops self-criticism and criticism of others one is in contact with. These introjections are expressed in the art work and in the way that the therapist is utilized in relation to creating art (Fairbairn, 1954).

Avital (D1) imagined herself as 'nothing', a white dot in a black page', which expresses the lack of formulation of self through not being 'seen' by her mother and thus of not being able to connect and then separate from her, and to become an individuated person.

Attachment styles

The dynamics of the primary relationships create styles of attachment, such as ambivalence (when the parent is ambivalent about the connection) anxiousness, disengagement, symbiosis, or security. These different styles of attachment will be manifest in art by drawn figures and in relationships, and projected on to the therapist (Bowlby, 1990).

Sharon (C1) drew although she did not want to because she was very 'good' and compliant, aiming to please the therapist and others in the group, but did not genuinely connect to anyone. This was apparent in her distant but neat stereotyped art — showing an ambivalent or 'false' type of attachment style.

Splits between 'good' versus 'bad' mother

Internalized relationships to the mother can also be split into different parts, such as extreme love and extreme anger towards the same parent, which cannot be integrated. This affects the ability to integrate one's personality and relationship with others. Art concretizes these splits and enables them to be visually integrated. They can also be expressed within the possibility of splitting between therapist and art work (Klein, 1932).

Rina (B1, B2) expressed splits in her art work between a colourful, perfect world, and a black, bad world, and in a woman split down the middle. These splits were also expressed in her behaviour of extreme niceness or extreme anger towards the therapist. Each side of the split was explored in the therapy and this enabled their integration.

Good enough mother

The gaps between reality and perfect attunement to the needs of others are the gaps that enable individuation from a symbiotic relationship with a parent in that the child learns to fill these gaps alone and still trust the parent. Lack of need fulfilment and too much need fulfilment are both detrimental to the process of individuation that eventually enable relationships with others that are not symbiotic. This can be expressed within art when the therapist is asked to 'guess' the meaning of the art, or to provide a perfect level of materials. Through the frustration of the art materials and interpretation as not being good enough, individuation is gradually enabled (Winnicott, 1958).

Avital (D 1) tested the therapist's ability to understand her 'white dot' and was disappointed that the therapist and group did not understand it as a self-portrait at the beginning. Gradually she accepted the need to explain her experience to herself and to others as a way to connect.

Transitional object

A transitional object is one that symbolically holds the qualities of the primary parent to enable separation from the primary object. Art work itself can be understood as such an object, as well as adult symbols such as religious artefacts, jewellery and wedding rings, which receive many relational projections.

> *Avital (D) made a small image of a plasticized heart for Rina to take with her when she felt she was going to enter into danger-seeking behaviour. This image became a transitional object for the positive power of the group for her, when she was not with the group (image not shown).*

Transitional space

Transitional space is the type of symbolic space created between people, which enables their working through different facets of relationships in a symbolic rather than direct way. Elements in the symbolic space can become reframed and changed through joint interaction. The symbolic spaces, in effect, enable both connection and individuation. For children, symbolic space is often in play and art work; and for adults often within cultural and work zones. Art therapy can be seen as a type of transitional space in itself (Winnicott, 1991).

> *The group as a whole created a transitional space using art that, on the one hand, 'illustrated' the group interactions, and on the other, enabled the group to address the shared sexual abuse indirectly and symbolically, entering and leaving different facets of the experience. The interaction between the art and the group created a 'double' symbolic, but also concrete, space for interpretation and change.*

Working the theory: art therapy skills and techniques

Verbal techniques

Verbal techniques include reflection on the way the client relates to the therapist, and to characters in their art work, and connection of this to early childhood relationships – as well as actively developing a different type of relationship with the therapist. (The client gradually trusts the art therapist to help with art materials without being invasive.) It might include reframing contents that prompt understanding, trust, and individuation. The role of the art therapist is therefore to use the art and relationship to understand, reflect, interpret, and correct object relations. Additionally, the aim is to actively create a transitional space in which relationships can be safely explored (Ainsworth, 1969; Bowlby, 1990; Coleman and

Farris-Dufrene, 1996; Fairbairn, 1954; Fishler *et al.*, 1990; Gomez, 1997; Higdon, 2004; Howard, 2006; Winnicott, 1958, 1991).

Visual techniques

Setting

The art therapist actively creates a playful, safe, and interactive zone that focuses on art making as a process rather than a product. The art's significance is that it is made in the context of the therapist's presence and interactive relationship. Another way of understanding this is through a safe setting that can be controlled or shared by the client, or therapist if this is what is needed, which promotes the possibility of play. The art setting and the relationship are in fact reciprocal.

Art process

The art process will focus on expressive, playful, and non-directive art being made in interaction with the observing art therapist, and on creative transitional spaces for interactive art games and processes. The focus in art making is on the creative expression that enables an exploration of different facets of the relationship, such as being separate, asking for help, being understood, or misunderstood, etc. The therapist can use his or her involvement to reframe the client's negative introjections (Dalley *et al.*, 1993; Malchiodi, 1998b; Robbins, 1999; Rubin, 1999).

Art interpretation

Art interpretation is based on analysing the interaction of client with therapist and projections on to the therapist and on to art. The art processes, products, and interpretations are used to understand introjected attachment styles and relationship issues. The dynamic gaps between words and art, and between content and composition, as well as between the use of therapist and use of page, are all analysed as potential expressions of unconscious conflicts, as explained in the previous chapter. For example, writing 'I love my mum' or 'my wife', in jagged disjointed lines with intense shading while being very angry with the female therapist may show ambivalent attachment in terms of the gaps between content and composition and interaction (Dalley *et al.*, 1993; Furth, 1998; Robbins, 1999; Rubin, 1999).

Overall skills to practise

* *Understanding one's own attachment styles*, introjected relationships and childhood experiences in order to monitor their interaction with those of the client.
* *Actively joining the client within the creation of transitional objects and transitional spaces*, within which relationships can be reflected and worked through. This means being able to interpret relationships by interacting with the client.

- *Reflecting and interpreting how attachment styles are expressed in interaction and in art*, but at the same time creating corrections within the zone of the relationship, for example, by gradually enabling more individuation and independent use of art, or conversely, providing a secure setting and help.
- *Encouraging projections on to self and on to objects* to create transitional objects and transitional spaces.
- *Encouraging expression of both positive and negative feelings* towards the drawn characters.

Art-based skills to practise

- Note transitional objects in your life (such as earrings, a handbag, etc.) and analyse their meanings for you.
- Create images of parents or primary caretakers, and try to understand attachment style and introjections through the image.
- Play a squiggle game or other interactive game with someone so as to learn to create a playful creative space together, and note your attachment style manifested in interaction.
- Watch children playing together and analyse their use of play to address relationships. Note when play 'fails'.
- Think of the symbolic transitional spaces within your own life, and create some if they are lacking.

Chapter 3

Art as the ego

Art therapy and ego psychology

The contribution of this theory to art therapy is that it suggests a proactive use of art as a tool for actively internalizing and practising more adaptive psychological reactions to conflicts. Many art therapy clients did not have the chance to develop these adaptive behaviours due to their environmental or neurological challenges, and art becomes a place that enables learning and internalization. This creates a theoretical base for using art in psychosocial interventions.

Ego-based theories, such as those developed by Anna Freud and Hartmann, focus on the ability of the ego to successfully mediate between id and superego and to solve inner conflicts (Freud 1936; Hartmann, 1964). Strengthening the ego becomes the focus of therapy. This includes a didactic element to therapy, in that people can learn to deal with inner conflicts through strengthening the ego. Some defences are more adaptive than others, and these can be actively modelled and strengthened.

The problem is thus defined as a weak ego that cannot utilize flexible and adaptive defences, and that cannot successfully negotiate the conflicts between id and superego.

The solution is to strengthen the ego and to integrate these more adaptive defences, such as sublimation, symbolization, and integration, instead of splitting, displacement, or dissociation. The therapist 'lends' his/her ego to the client and models adaptive defences and positive negotiation between id and superego (Ainsworth, 1969; Freud, 1936; Goldstein, 1995; Hartmann, 1964; Higdon, 2004).

As stated in Chapter 2, the social context of Anna Freud's work was the focus on childhood as being separate from adulthood (Higdon, 2004). The role of education as strengthening the emotional integrity and developing ego is central to the more optimistic focus, possibly also reflecting the times.

Macro applications include a belief in a community's abilities to strengthen its collective 'ego' by learning more adaptive ways to resolve conflicts and traumas through utilizing more flexible defences, such as sublimation. For example, a community can move from satisfying immediate needs by throwing refuse in a public place, to creating a recycled playground with the rubbish; or a community can create a commemorative sculpture to express loss of loved ones in the war, rather than suffering individually (Howard, 2006; Mitchell, 1995; Wolfgang, 2006).

The role of art from this perspective is understood not only as located within the id, and as a projection and catharsis of basic drives, but also as located within the ego, which can channel basic energy into symbolic, integrated, sublimated responses to inner conflicts and painful experiences. This enables a more proactive role for art. Art making, and all symbolic interaction, is a zone for decision making, containment of strong emotions, and integration of experience. Art enables processes of containment, sublimation, clarification, and compromise, when it emerges from the ego. Art also encourages regression, but because of this, it helps the client to move beyond regression to adaptive developmental problem solving as in regression in the service of the ego. The focus shifts from analysis of the product to working with the process of art making and evaluating its psychological quality. Thus art moves from an expression of unconscious conflicts to an attempt to psychologically address these conflicts. There is a correlation between psychological quality and aesthetic quality, in that complex psychological processes within art will render a complex and high-quality art product (Ball, 2002; Case and Daley, 1990; Coleman and Farris-Dufrene, 1996; Heegaard, 2001; Kramer, 1971, 2000; Malchiodi, 1998a; Stepney, 2001; Wadeson, 2000).

The role of the art therapist is to encourage the client to express conflicts, and also to utilize more adaptive coping mechanisms in relation to these conflicts. Projections, transferences, and interpretations are still the frame, but also encouragement of reactions that contain sublimation, integration, and containment of emotions help the client learn to utilize more adaptive defences and strategies. The therapist, as it were, 'joins' the client's ego, lending his or her own strengths, and as such is also a teacher and guide. The above adaptive coping strategies are modelled and enacted within the art making. Interpretations are offered in relation to the evolving art process, rather than directly; art solutions are used to model more adaptive psychological solutions and insight on a preconscious level. The art therapist is thus also an art teacher, and a role model of adaptive solutions.

Art evaluation is based on the use and development of more adaptive and flexible defence mechanisms, as expressed in process and quality of art making, which is generalized to behaviour and overall sense of self. Art evaluation techniques include a focus on the psychological mechanisms used while making art and their manifestation in the art process, composition, and product. Kramer provides a typology of art according to defences that includes stereotypical art, that is a defence against real feelings, lack of integration in art, as shown in the compositional elements, and the gradual process of reaching sublimated and integrative art products that will show a high-quality art depiction. Thus, the process and product will show the types of defences used (Kramer, 1971; 2000).

Supervision will be based on understanding the art processes as different types of defences and on thinking how to encourage more adaptive use of the ego through additional art techniques and processes. Transferences and relationships will be addressed but the aim will be to situate the projections within the art processes.

The research will be hermeneutically oriented through a case study, focusing on the creation of art works and on their transformation (Case and Daley, 1990; Kramer, 1971). Conversely, the ways that defences are expressed as well as modified within art works will be researched (Kramer, 1971).

A possible critique of this theory is that it assumes that problems are based in a weak ego, rather than in inherent difficulties (e.g. learning difficulties) or in extreme social problems (e.g. lack of resources). Another assumption is that these processes in art will be generalized to life.

Central concepts exemplified through case study

Symbolization and sublimation

These concepts are more socially adept methods of using art to deal with difficult feelings, and demand cognitive and emotional skills that enable the use of complex symbols as containers, definers, and reframers of emotions.

> Shoshana (A1) started with a page of blackness, and gradually found words to better symbolize her feelings. The black hole has become a more communicative and nuanced symbol of the woman's painful experience and hints at more positive qualities in the 'world'.

Integration

The ability to integrate rather than split or dissociate or polarize conflicting emotions is central to being able to adjust to people as good and bad, loving and angry, etc. Art visually concretizes the integration of opposing emotions into the same gestalt.

> Rina (B1, B2) shifted from pictures split between white and black, or split down the middle, to images that integrated colour and blackness. (B3, B4). Her behaviour also became more accepting and modulated in the group and she stopped getting into high-risk situations and left her high-risk boyfriend.

Sublimation

This is considered an effective and positive defence.

> Avital (D2) managed to express her anger at her mother's lack of protection in red oil pastel contained within a black shape. This was a sublimated example of her anger that did not harm her or others, or overwhelm her because it was contained within a symbol. Thus she as 'nothing' (D1) was replaced by herself full of red anger (D2). After this, she created flowers as colourful rich circles (D3). This gradual shift reflects her sublimation of and integration of anger through her art.

Working the theory: art therapy skills and techniques

Verbal techniques

These will focus on reflection and on interpretation but also on modelling and suggesting explanations within the art that reflect psychological solutions within flexible understandings and use of defences (Higdon, 2004).

Visual techniques

Setting

The setting will provide high-quality art products and easels to enable ongoing art work, to encourage more elaborate and process-oriented art. This type of art enables the formation of integrative symbols, and deep containment of an expression of difficult emotions. Careful choice and use of art techniques and materials may foster these expressions. For example, the use of high-quality acrylic or oil paints enables the layering of levels of paint, symbolizing the layering and integration of meanings. Having good quality clay and glazes enables them to be fired, thus creating a higher quality product – as higher sublimation of primary drives – than by just using clay and letting it air dry.

Process

The art therapist will use knowledge of art as well as therapy to provide the right technique and material for presenting the psychological issue within art processes. The process will aim to create a high-quality art product that can be held and actively guided by the therapist. The art therapist may use her knowledge of materials and art, as well as her knowledge of dynamic processes. The art therapist will aim to 'join' the client's ego in actualizing an image from his or her head on to the page, which may include modulating frustration and self-destruction (e.g. painting so hard that the page tears).

Interpretation

Interpretation will be ongoing in terms of addressing and trying to enhance the quality of defences used and translating them into the art making. The therapist will translate these psychological processes into comments upon the art processes and products, encouraging sublimation, articulation, and integration. The interpretation can stay within the art process and product or can be interpreted back to the therapist's life (Ball, 2002; Case and Daley, 1990; Coleman and Farris-Dufrene, 1996; Heegaard, 2001; Kramer, 1971, 2000; Malchiodi, 1988; Stepney, 2001; Wadeson, 2000).

Overall skills to practise

- *The ability to interpret according to meta-theory*, the defences, regressions and conflicts expressed within the art and to translate these into art activities that encourage more adaptive defences.
- *Art skills and techniques*. Knowledge of art materials and techniques and artists as well as experience of artistic processes (artist identity) so as to be able to suggest complex art processes that can translate effective integration and sublimation of primary drives into art products.
- *Ability to contain client's frustration and to model adaptive ways* of dealing with frustration, pain, flooding, depression, translated into art behaviour. This demands an ability to work with one's own defences and to keep them flexible and adaptive in relation to the client.

Art-based skills to practise

- Conflicts: take a conflict that you feel strongly about and try to create an integrative image of it.
- Transitions and loss: create an art work that becomes a commemoration for a lost person, place or state; work on it until the feeling is truly 'held' by the art.
- Coping with childhood pain: try to express an old anger in an abstract art work, and then to turn it into an additional symbol.
- Create a portrait of someone problematic in your life, try to locate and to express the complex feelings this person arouses in you, while also being able to show the person itself.

Chapter 4

Culturally contextualized art as healing on a preconscious level

Art therapy and Jung

Jungian theory has a strong contribution to art therapy at the level of its focus on the deep connection between people and the visual world around them, and on the healing power of engaging with art even at a preconscious level, that is, without a therapist. This can be seen as the root of the art as therapy conception. This challenges various paradigms in art therapy, pointing to the need to work within the symbolic construct and experiences of a specific culture, and to expand art therapy to include a broader definition of visual culture.

Jungian theory claims that in addition to an individual unconscious, people have a collective unconscious that is expressed through different symbols within each culture. These culturally contextualized symbols hold a collective unconscious comprised of experiences and past traumas of the group. They also contain different depictions of the same basic universal archetypes that are expressed in similar compositional elements in all cultures. Examples of such archetypes include the persona or the external self we use in society, the anima, which is the sexual, gendered self; and the shadow, which depicts the dark and aggressive self. According to this, cultural symbols are a place in which people work through inner conflicts on preconscious levels by projecting on to archetypes that are accessible as culturally contextualized symbols. This theory is a shift away from Freud both at the level of the connection created between the individual and society as expressed within culture, and at the more optimistic, preconscious level of people being able to resolve their own conflicts. The broad revelatory character of socially contextualized, multi-sensory symbols enables the reconnection to archetypes and through this, the projection, containment, and reinterpretation of personal experience.

A problem is defined when people cannot work through their inner conflicts with the help of socially contextualized archetypes. One solution is to reconnect to symbols and cultural art activities that enable the preconscious integration of inner conflicts (Fontana, 1993; Jung, 1974).

One can understand the social context of Jung's theory through the colonialist setting that bought artefacts from many different cultures, and which fascinated the intellectual elite (Edwards, 2001; Howard, 2006).

The macro application of Jung's theory expands the intra-psychic theories of Freud to include a cultural component. Jung helped to connect between people and society. Thus, in sociological terms, a theory such as symbolic interaction – or in dynamic terms, projection on to cultural symbols – enables the individual to reorient and reintegrate his/her personal conflicts within his/her visual culture. At the social level of rehabilitation, art therefore has the potential to be a self-initiated, culturally contextualized method of community healing, which is based in restoring symbols of meaning that help reorganize community solidarity and resilience through enabling individuals to undertake the intra-psychic work of psychological healing. Examples are taken from the experience of the persecution of the holocaust, or the slavery of African people, as a trauma within the psyche of all of these ethnic groups – even for those who did not experience it directly. The symbols connected to these experiences arouse strong emotions in all members of these groups and become symbols through which to attribute meaning to individual problems.

The role of art is central to this theory, and focuses on visual symbols as the arena where internal archetypes are manifested. Art's role shifts to a culturally contextualized mediator between individual and collective experience, through symbols. Art helps to mediate between the unconscious and preconscious levels of experience (Jung, 1974). This definition of art expands from dreams and fine art to include ritualistic and religious art, crafts, and cultural icons within a given society. The assumption is thus that art is healing, through connection to meaningful symbols. From this, the cultural symbolic forms of expression that surround us gain a social and psychological role of self-regulation of inner conflicts (Edwards, 2001; Furth, 1998). Art becomes a therapeutic medium in its own right, in that cultural symbols are able to 'hold' emotions and to help transform them – not neccesarily with the intervention of a therapist. If in Freudian theory the content level is the conscious level, and the compositional level is the unconscious level, then here the content level is the culturally contextualized symbol and the compositional level contains the unconscious universal archetypes of the self (Edwards, 2001; Furth, 1998; Jung, 1974; Wesley, 2008; Wilson, 2001). For example, all types of religions have a circular mandala-like shape that symbolizes the whole and transcendent self: similarly, all cultures have symbols of 'shadows' that depict the aggressive and darker self.

Another central role of the art therapist, in addition to all of the dynamic skills previously described, is to pay attention to projection, transference and counter-transference, defences, and childhood stages that are unable to develop (see Chapter 2). The Jungian art therapist also practises interpretation of the client's images and symbols in dreams, fantasies, and narratives according to the archetypes that they contain in relation to the client's current conflict. Another new and major role is to encourage the client to engage in creativity, or in projection on to cultural symbols, to utilize them towards a preconscious healing of conflicts. The therapist's assumption is that engaging the client with dreams, art, or other symbolic elements in their life, becomes part of the self-healing process, also at a preconscious level, through creative engagement with symbols that contain meaningful archetypes. The focus shifts from the relationship with the therapist to engagement with creativity (although both are still used) (Edwards, 2001; Furth, 1998; Jung, 1974; Wesley, 2008; Wilson, 2001).

Working the theory: art therapy skills and techniques

Verbal techniques

As covered in Chapter 3, verbal techniques include the use of free association, dreams, jokes, and also active focus on other images and symbols that the client raises in his narratives, with the inclusion of the meta-theory of symbols and archetypes, and the collective unconscious, through which to interpret contents. Theories of introvert-extrovert personality can also be used. Cultural symbols and archetypes are analysed in relation to the client's specific conflicts and problems.

Visual techniques

The focus will shift to creating meaningful art symbols that are healing in themselves in that even without interpretation they enable the working through of preconscious conflicts. It can include a joint deciphering of the meaning of a symbol and its archetype by therapist and client. In other words, the therapist and client both actively focus on the art.

The setting

The art setting often includes a focus on ready-made art products (e.g. various materials and images such as magazine pictures depicting existing images or symbols) in order to enhance the client's visual engagement with them. This makes the setting more like a studio than a 'blank screen' neutral environment. Meaningful images may be exhibited or hung up for further contemplation and different depictions of archetypes can be compared and observed.

The art processes

The overall dynamic focus on free art expression remains, but shifts to encouraging creativity and engagement with symbols as an inherently healing activity. The overall focus therefore shifts from projections on to the therapist, and expression of conflicts, to creative engagement with images. The art therapist can use directed engagement with ritualistic, religious, and craft icons, which hold universal archetypes within cultural forms. For example, a client might describe the emotional impact for him of seeing images of mandalas in churches, and the therapist could encourage him to draw a mandala that expresses the client's search for self at present; or a teenager could discuss the 'vampire' movies that he loves, the vampire being drawn as a 'shadow archetype', and developed in relation to the client's own shadows.

The integration of the archetype occurs within four discrete stages: (a) familiarization with the unconscious contents found in the art work; (b) acknowledgement or 'ownership' of these contents, rather than their denial; (c) assimilation, or working through the meaning of this symbolism into reality; and (d) disposal. This is the last stage and once it has been done, the client will not need the image any more. This intense process as a whole makes the art work or symbolic content *'embodied'*, that is, full of projections and meaning (Schaverien, 1999).

Art analysis

As stated, the analysis is less important than the emotional engagement with art symbols. Analysis includes identifying and paying attention to recurring symbols within the client's art, and to compositional archetypes that the symbols embody, in terms of the client's current conflicts in life (Robbins, 1999; Schaverien, 1999). For example, the circular repetitive mandala shape, which expresses the harmonious self and is apparent in all cultures, is the symbol of integration, harmony, and perfection. It helps us strive to be our best selves in harmony with the world, and to integrate different facets of self. This wholeness usually occurs within midlife, rather than in youth.

The shadow is the dark, evil, or sadistic side of the personality which is the reason for cruelty. Admitting and identifying symbols of the shadow helps to deal with it. The shadow symbol is identified by its darkness: the persona, or outward mask, is how we describe ourselves to society, and is defined by how others expect us to be. This shadow symbol becomes negative when we identify too much with our persona, but it is a way of understanding social roles within society. The anima and animus are symbols of characteristics of the opposite sex that might include, for example in women, the witch, prostitute, goddess, mother; and in men, the hero, adventurer, or villain.

Evaluation

According to this theory evaluation will cover transference, interpretation of defences, and stuck (calcified) childhood stages as in all dynamic therapy. Art evaluation is based on levels of emotional immersion in symbols and on the relief gained from this preconscious engagement of content in the symbols and their archetypes in the context of the client's specific issues.

Supervision

Supervision will not only focus on the general frame of transference and countertransference, but also on deciphering the client's central symbolic formations in terms of archetypes and personal development. Supervision will also encourage clients in ways that will prompt the preconscious to work through issues (e.g. encouraging the client to look at symbols that seem important to her at present and then to create art from them) (Simon, 2005; Wilson, 2001).

Research

According to the Jungian meta-theory, research may take the form of a case study, focusing on how people utilize archetypal and cultural symbols to resolve problems, based on their personality type. Another direction might be cultural and social, typifying different universal and cultural symbols within a social context. This can intersect with anthropological and cultural theories, as well as with today's visual culture (Moon, 2008).

Critique

A central critique of Jung can be the colonialist assumption of universality of archetypes in all cultures, that is, Western psychology is relevant to all (Mitchell, 1995; Mohanty, 2003; Said, 1978). The archetypes and personality orientations may also create a somewhat rigid and narrow theory of conflicts. The general direction points to a highly functioning client interested in self-fulfilment and creativity enhancement, rather than suffering from acute symptoms or social stress (Schultz and Schultz, 2011).

Central concepts exemplified through case study

Symbols

As stated, symbols are culturally constructed at the level of content and specific form within each culture, but are also manifestations of universal archetypes at the level of composition. By definition symbols hold an intense cluster of meanings that are both dynamic and shifting. They can be found in cultural artefacts, and in dreams and images of the individual.

> *All of the women (ABCD) used a black shape as a symbol of the sexual abuse that they had suffered, which can be seen as a collective symbol that included the archetype of the 'shadow'.*

The collective unconscious

This is the pool of cultural symbols and experiences through which the individual does the above-mentioned therapeutic work: it is connected to the cultural group that the client belongs to.

> *Shoshana (A2) used words from a traditional Israeli song that is part of the collective unconscious about how unjust the world is.*

Archetypes

Archetypes are universal constructs that are compositionally similar, and can be found within central cultural symbols.

Rina (B2, B3,) created a mandala shape of 'self' when she managed to integrate her former dissociated splits. Sharon (C2, C4) also shifted to mandala-like doodles expressing her gradual meeting with 'self'.

Familiarization, acknowledgement, assimilation, and disposal

We see that Shoshana (D1) first became familiar with her expression of self as a white hole with no content. She then owned this experience of lack of identity and was angry, assimilating her emotions into her next image of red circles (D2), and then disposed of the images within her large poster where they were unrecognizable (D3).

Overall skills to practise

- *Actively engaging with cultural symbols of one's own culture* and learning to look for archetypes within symbols.
- *Learning to look for symbols and archetypes in other cultures* (those of clients).
- *Listening for visual symbols within the client's narratives,* and encouraging them to be drawn or visualized, to identify the archetypes within the symbol.
- *Encouraging the client's engagement with creative processes,* which can include art making but also engagement in cultural activities that are expressed with symbols, such as going to a play or engaging with religious symbols, or watching a film or television.
- *Identifying and encouraging the stages of familiarization, acknowledgement, assimilation, and disposal* in relation to the client's art process.

Art-based skills to practise

- Searching for and identifying culturally conceptualized symbols and their compositional archetypes within one's own art work and relating to present issues.
- Searching for meaningful symbols within day-to-day visual culture, and analysing them in terms of archetypes and personal life.
- Keeping a dream diary and a sketchbook and noting recurring dreams.
- Gathering images of central symbols in your culture to work on with clients.

Summary of dynamic theories

We have seen that dynamic theories focus on the difference between content and composition: for Freud, content is consciousness, and composition is unconscious; for Jung content is culture, and composition is the universal problems of the psyche; for Winnicott, content and composition are interactive zones where inner and outer reality can meet; and for ego psychology, content is an expression of the power of the ego, as shown in Table 4.1.

We have seen that although all of these theories utilize the dynamic meta-theory, they interpret it in different ways, which creates many understandings of the art therapy components: these differences have been summarized in Table 4.2.

Table 4.1 Dynamic theories: content, composition, and role of therapist

	Content	*Composition*	*Therapist*
Dynamic	Conscious	Unconscious	Interpreter of id
Ego psychology	Conscious	Unconscious processes	Encourager of adaptive processes that integrate composition and content
Object relationship	Conscious elements of relationship	Unconscious elements of relationship	Initiator of interactive space
Jung	Cultural, conscious	Universal psyche, unconscious	Interpreter of symbols and archetypes

Table 4.2 Comparison of dynamic theories

	Freudian	Object relations	Ego psychology	Jungian theory
Setting	Neutral to encourage projections	Playful enabling interaction between therapist and client	Art studio set up with variety of quality materials	Includes ready-made images of symbols and art materials
Art process	Undirected by therapist	Can be interactive between therapist and client	Adaptive psychological mechanisms are encouraged in relation to art processes	Focus on symbols and hidden archetypes in client's narratives, dreams, and art work
Art product	Interpreted according to meta-theory of defences and conflicts	Interpreted as unconscious introjections of attachment	Interpreted as expression of a psychological process	Interpreted as holding archetype of issue within symbol
Therapist's role	Uses reflection and interpretation of relationship and art interactively; neutral stance	Creates interaction with client around art that reflects relationship	Models and encourages art techniques that enable integrative expressive and sublimated art processes	Encourages engagement with symbols that hold meaningful archetypes for client
Art evaluation	Evaluation of insight reached through content of art as conscious and composition is as unconscious material	Evaluation of shifts in internalized relationships shown in art interaction and product	Art is evaluated according to quality of defences and psychological processing that are manifest in quality of art	Evaluation of use of archetypes within symbols as psychological resources
Supervision	Focus on parallel processes between therapist and supervisor and deciphering unconscious materials in art	Focus on relationship and on creating transitional space	Focus on translating psychological processes into art processes	Focusing on deciphering symbols and archetypes and on utilizing them for client development
Research	Quantifiable compositional elements as reflection of conflicts or hermeneutic case studies	Case studies of interaction between client and therapist as expressed in art work. Analyses of attachment styles within interaction and art product	Includes how different defences are depicted in art, as well as descriptions of art processes that embody psychological processes	Case studies of use of archetypes and symbols and typologies of cultural symbols and their archetypes

B

ART AS A PATH TO THE SELF THROUGH UNCONDITIONAL ACCEPTANCE: INTRODUCTION TO HUMANISTIC THEORIES

Humanistic and positive psychology theories focus on the inherent uniqueness, individuality, and potential of each person. Everyone can blossom when they have the core conditions of unconditional acceptance, respect, and fulfilment of basic needs; and, if taught to handle stress effectively, one can focus on the positive and on self-regulation according to positive psychology theories.

Art becomes a zone in which to explore meaning and to reach an authentic self, a place to visualize positive outcomes, or ability to self-actualize. Art is interpreted by the artist-client as his/her subjective experience or perception of reality. Thus, creativity becomes an encompassing and individual process. Art also becomes a zone in which to create meaning and to reframe meanings, in existential and narrative theories, to connect to one's experiences and to integrate different facets of experience according to gestalt theories. Art symbolically expresses and strengthens developmental challenges over a lifetime according to developmental theories. Art therefore becomes a path not to the unconscious, but to the authentic self.

The focus is on process and on how the product is interpreted, rather than on the product as separate from the client and interpreted by a dynamic meta-theory, as in the dynamic theories. The phenomenological experience of self and of life is accessed, expressed, shared, and reorganized through art. A problem does not have the core conditions that enable this process of exploration of self, and the solution is to create and to identify those conditions and the evolving self, through art engagement. Art is an active way to define and focus on the positive potential; it is a holistic way to connect between mind, body, emotions, and soul, and it is a physical way to create self-regulation. While these vital and central roles for art point to art as 'healing' in itself, it is important to remember that these roles are only relevant within the context of the overall humanistic theory, otherwise artists would be inherently psychologically and physically healthy. In fact, within the context of the fine art world, art is a stressful, often false effort to impress others.

The variations within this theory are outlined in the following diagram and will be explored within this section:

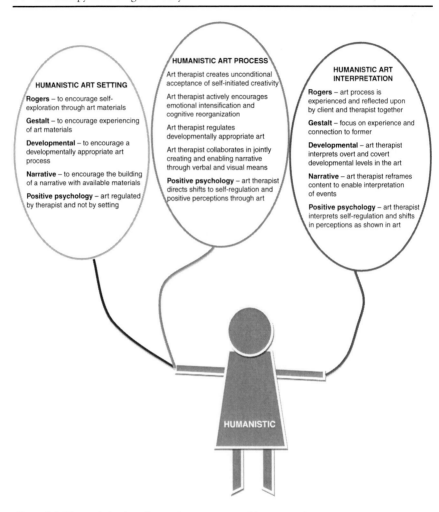

Figure 5.1 Humanistic theories: setting, process, and interpretation

Chapter 5

Art as a path to the self
Art therapy and humanistic theories

Contributions of humanistic theory are central to art therapy as they provide a central role for art, as an inherent and self-directed creative process, which leads to self-knowledge and to self-fulfilment in a positive, flexible, and enabling way. Art is given a principal role in humanity, as a path to self-knowledge and to self-actualization. Art becomes 'healing' in the context of the core conditions of unconditional acceptance of the art therapist.

Humanistic theories diverge from dynamic theories in that they conceive of people as being able to access their unconscious, and to regulate and decipher their own lives as an ongoing process. At each stage this processing provides them with new opportunities for self-actualization. Humanistic theories are based on a belief in people's inherent goodness, authenticity, individuality, and inherent drive towards self-fulfilment if given the core conditions, or right emotional climate to enable this development. The inherent uniqueness and drive towards self-fulfilment of each person is the strongest therapeutic force. This stance is informed by philosophical existential and phenomenological theories that elaborate upon humanity's ability to utilize free choice and to create subjective meaning, based on the fact that we have to bear the eventual inevitable end of life – and, according to existential philosophy that highlights free will and phenomenology, there is no divine force that can guide us except ourselves. A person's psychological state will depend on the meanings that he/she attributes to life events: at the relationship level, as described in the object theories, the 'core conditions' of fulfilment of basic needs, respect, and non-judgemental acceptance are what enable the person to accept herself and her own authentic core. This can be found at different stages of life, in different relationships, with each stage able to correct former negative experiences. Therapy not only searches for unconscious elements, but includes the whole person as a single and interactive organism, made up of the interconnected physical, social, spiritual, and psychological facets of self (Frankl, 1985; Maslow, 1970; Mearns and Thomas, 2007; Rogers, 1995).

Problems may be defined as being based in the huge responsibility of individuals to explain their life's meaning on account of free will, as well as a lack of the core conditions of acceptance, respect, and fulfilment of the basic needs that are necessary for self-actualization.

The solution is to actively create a context of self-acceptance and genuineness, and to find core conditions that enable development. The ability of people to create their own destiny is therefore not only the problem but also the solution, as we are able to perceive and understand life events in a way that is meaningful to us (Butler, 2001; Frankl, 1985; Misiak, 1973).

This theory was created during the post-world war social context of financial affluence and optimism in the USA. This context enabled people to concentrate on self-actualization rather than on survival, or the counter-culture of decline of the grand theories, and power of the state after the wars (including the Vietnam War) (DeCarvalho, 1991; Elkins, 2008). The humanistic values were strongly situated within progressive educational movements of the time, where art was considered a central educational and developmental tool for children's cognitive as well as emotional development (Gardner, 1993; Hansen, 2001; Hills 2001; Johnson, 1999; Lowenfield, 1987). In the USA, these directions were parallel to current scientific and behaviourist views that focused on measuring shifts in observable and 'objective' behaviour, rather than in experiences of behaviour (Leary, 1994; Sokal, 1984).

Macro applications focus on the subjective legitimization of the individual, which includes all individuals regardless of race or class. This can be seen as a social stance that humanizes all sectors of society, as well as institutions and settings, where individual experience and legitimacy are questioned. The authentic experience of a group and ways that communities create meaning together can also be related to this theory. Rogers defines society or 'core conditions' of basic respect as central for psychological growth (Rogers, 1995). It can be argued that people coping with the most basic levels of Maslow's pyramid also have souls, potential, dreams, and deserve the right to self-actualize, to make meaning out of their reality. Holding on to a holistic humanism of all types of populations is a way to address racism and social injustice, and thus a tool for fighting marginalization.

The role of art is therefore defined as a way of expressing and creating meaning, and as a way of facilitating dialogue with the self and others. Authentic experience replaces unconscious experience, which can be accessed through creative pursuits. Art as self-expression in Western culture is a natural field for existentialism because art itself creates meaning and gives meaning to life. It is also inherently phenomenological as it enables the individual to express and thus access her authentic feelings and individuality. Everyone is potentially creative and the central 'artist' of her own life. As stated, in continuation of this, art becomes a central tool in education and has a crucial role in society (Gardner, 1993; Lowenfield, 1987).

Taking this further, the role of the art therapist is to enable creative self-expression because authentic activity is understood by the art therapist to be psychologically important without relation to the level of art created, or to the interpretation or intervention of the therapist. The client is the definer of the meaning and value of the art, rather than an external art or psychology expert (compared to fine art, where the critic is the central authority), or dynamic diagnostic art, where the psychologist is the central authority. Composition and content become tools through which the artist can access his authentic inner self (Cooper, 2008; Higdon, 2004;

Yalom, 1994). The art therapist is responsible for creating the core conditions of acceptance, encouragement, and enablement of the above process. The therapist's development of an 'artist identity' through constant self-art is based on the assumption that one cannot encourage creativity in others without developing creativity in oneself as an ongoing discipline (McNiff, 1998; Moon, 2002; Robbins, 1999; Rogers, 1993; Silverstone, 1993). The humanistic theory is at the base of counselling techniques that often provide the theoretical frame for art therapy, as found in the USA (Rubin, 2001).

Therapy evaluation is assessed collaboratively by the client and therapist, based on the subjective experience of progress and on the quality of relationship and self-expression. This is an ongoing process that does not reach a set conclusion, although symptoms of stress and self-destructive behaviours will be assumed to be reduced through deeper self-actualization. Because these processes are subjective, they cannot be defined or measured outside of the client's own subjective terms. This might include getting in touch with past pain and sadness – not just improvements in symptoms in humanistic theories – while in positive psychology the focus is on shifts to positive and enabling narratives, rather than a focus on the past.

Art-based evaluations will focus on overall communication, creativity, authenticity, and expressivity of art use rather than on the product. It will evaluate if and how the art has become an arena through which the client expresses and gets to know the self.

Supervision will focus on the relationship, on efforts to provide core conditions of authentic non-judgemental trust and respect towards the client, and ways to help this occur through a parallel modelled relationship with the supervisor. The therapist's art work can be used as a method to explore the therapist's feelings towards the client and vice versa. The client's overall process will be discussed and conceptualized.

Research will be based on a phenomenological description of case studies and on collaborative description of the client's own self-described processes (Allen, 1995; Silverstone, 1993). The explosion in qualitative and art-based methods of research, especially in education, is based on the humanistic premise that subjective experience and personal interpretation are central to understanding the research participants, rather than using predetermined issues defined by researchers (Eisner, 1997; Foster, 2007; Gilroy, 2006; Huss, 2012a; Knowles and Cole, 2008).

A possible critique of the humanistic approach is that it is elitist because it implies potential free choice for everyone; it ignores the reality of socially marginalized groups. In terms of art and creativity, these may seem like luxuries for populations dealing with marginalization, basic survival, or other extreme symptoms. In terms of the relationships, the assumption that the therapist can be genuine and create an authentic relationship might also seem somewhat naïve when working with extreme defences. Additionally, in terms of cultural relevance, the therapist's concept of self-expression and creativity as expression of self is based on Western art uses, and is not part of the aesthetic language of many groups, including working-class Western groups. From this, then, the romantic concept of art as spontaneous and 'health inducing', or art as ' medicine', which are often thrown around in art therapy, is problematic in that it assumes that Western creativity is healing for all people. In addition to ignoring social theories, therefore, the theory also ignores cultural and psychological realities that may include defences against traumatic situations that do not enable the flexibility or self-directedness needed for this type of creativity. It is a critique most suited to middle-class Western populations as a form of self-exploration, rather than addressing the deep social or psychological suffering of many groups (Kvale, 1992; Leary, 1994; Miller, 1996).

Central concepts exemplified through case study

Core conditions

Core conditions include the unconditional self-acceptance and genuineness of the therapist towards the client in verbal and art interactions. The non-judgemental presence of the therapist, and the open non-directive setting in which individuals can express themselves, are essential for creative expression, and through that, self-actualization.

> *The art therapist created core conditions by accepting and not judging the need of the women to create very controlled repetitive designs at the beginning of the group. She did not interpret this or suggest moving to more expressive materials but accepted it as an authentic expression of their reality. Avital (D) did not draw at all for the first few months and this was respected as a form of self-expression congruent to her experience at the time.*

Authentic self

People search for their authentic inner self. Self-expression is the process that enables this journey, and is synonymous with the emergence of the inner individual and 'authentic' self.

> *Sharon started off drawing to please the therapist as is seen in the disconnected character of her art. Gradually her doodles became more centred and expressive, as she found her authentic self (3A, 3B, 3D).*

Pyramid of needs

Art as a physical, emotional, and cognitive activity enables the different parts of self to be integrated. Maslow ordered these different levels into a triangle, pointing to the physical needs as basic, but reducing compared to emotional and spiritual needs. Although a person may experience poverty and physical needs, the assumption is that they also have emotional and spiritual needs that if addressed, will help create the strength to cope with fulfilling basic physical needs.

Shoshana (A) first had to connect to her dream of having a child in order to find the energy to deal with the physical fear of medical intervention involved with fertility. The image of her authentic wish for a child (A4) enabled her to connect to her higher levels of values and aspirations and to find the strength to confront her physical fear.

Engaging with art for personal insight

Betinsky's method is for the client to engage with her own art work and address the composition to explore levels of meaning, which are interpreted by the client rather than the therapist enabling the client to reach new levels of authentic self (Betinsky, 1995).

Rina looked at her art work and could clearly see the splits that she employed within the compositions of her images (B1, B2). These images are a type of dialogue with her defences through art, as shown in her gradual efforts to integrate the split in B3 and B4.

Existential search for meaning

The individual needs to face the anxiety, uncertainty, meaninglessness, and eventual end of life. Art becomes a way to deal with finding one's meaning and place in the world.

Avital (D3) found meaning for her suffering by creating a poster of images and using it to better the situation of other women who had undergone sexual abuse.

Free will and the potential for self-actualization

In contrast to Freudian theories that say that people are directed by the unconscious, humanistic theory understands people as being directed primarily by their free will. This enables self-actualization, as already described, but also puts responsibility on the individual, rather than on fate, society, or unconscious drives. Within art the client can direct and choose the contents. The empty page can be understood as a zone of free will.

Shoshana replaced the blackness, symbolizing her abuse, at the centre of her life (or image) in her first images (A1, A2, A3) gradually giving the black less prominence on the page and focusing more on the other colours. With an image of a baby instead of blackness at the centre of her continuing image (A4), she used her free will and ability to create meaning in her life to negate the impact of her traumatic experience on her future life.

Working the theory: art therapy skills and techniques

Verbal techniques

The therapist aims to create an authentic, person-to-person encounter and to encourage the client to listen to herself and to define her own meanings through absence of judgement, encouragement, kindness, respect, safety, and concern that stems from genuine interest in the client. These become the core conditions needed for the client's self-actualization. The therapist achieves this transformation by utilizing his authentic self as an active witness, rather than by judging, interpreting, or initiating change in the client. In other words, the meeting with the therapist is understood not only as projective (as in dynamic theories) but also as a new and corrective meeting in the present. The therapist connects meaninglessness and isolation to create new social, psychological, physical, and spiritual meanings, rather than explore past developmental problems. In general, this concept of therapy as a meeting between two authentic people shifts the notion of a therapist from a clinician to a 'person'. A person might meet many therapeutic figures in a lifetime who provide unconditional and accepting support of her individuality, such as religious leaders, or other friends that help us through crises.

The therapist uses feedback, reflection, reframing, and encouragement rather than interpretation, confrontation, or a 'blank screen' persona. The therapist must strive to discourage transference and counter-transference by focusing on the real person in the present – and on the potential for a corrective relationship. She strives to address her own need to judge and lack of acceptance of the client through supervision, and searches for genuine, respectful responses (Cooper, 2008; Higdon, 2004; Yalom, 1994).

Visual techniques

Setting

The therapist will aims to create an enabling, self-directed setting that is calm, inviting, and flexible. Materials are diverse, and controlled by the client, encouraging exploration of different sensations and experiences. The client decides if the art will be personal, or public. The studio becomes a self-actualizing zone, enabling non-judgemental use of materials, responsibility towards one's own process, and freedom of choice (Allen, 1995; McNiff, 1998; Moon, 2003, 2008).

Art process

The client is in charge of choosing materials and contents and the therapist is a helpful witness but does not direct the art process. The therapist's reactions to the art created can include genuine feedback, focused on respect and enablement, as well as encouragement for further self-exploration through additional art making. The therapist may also utilize his own creativity to help the client along the path she has chosen, offering encouragement and suggestions rather than directives. The therapist aims to provide authentic reactions to the art. For example, the therapist might tell the client how moving it was to watch her struggle to find the right colour to express her emotion, and struggle to overcome her self-criticism at the level of the product (using feedback). The art therapist may see a client very upset and suggest hanging up a large page and using paints to capture that feeling – but the client will decide, it will not be presented as a directive but as a possibility. The focus is on enhancing emotional connectedness rather than on cognitive understanding of the art process.

Art interpretation

The client and therapist together think of meanings with which to analyse the images; or not analyse it but think of additional art activities to further explore the issues. Emotional connection may be the aim rather than formal analyses of meaning, similar to Jung's assumption that art enables healing on a preconscious level. Both process and product are analysed on the same level; most importantly, the interpretation is based on the phenomenological experiences of the client, and not on an interpretive meta-theory of the therapist. The analyses are thus collaborative, and art is used to gain further insight into themes that resonate for the client. The shifts between art work and interpretation, and then more art work to explore the themes that the client identified, are ongoing.

In terms of art analyses, Betinsky outlines a method where the therapist leads the client to concentrate carefully on the composition of the image, and to reach insights into its meaning with his help. This is different from the therapist analysing the compositional elements according to a pre-existing meta-theory as in dynamic theory, but instead is based on the client's intense connection and exploration of her art and on her intuitive ability to reach her own understanding (Betinsky, 1995). Allen also developed a method of 'intentionality' in which a person can decide to focus on an issue in her mind, and then let the art lead her to insights and exploration of the issue. Again, the concept is that the ability to access meaning is in the client's power (Allen, 1995). Moon and others also focus on the 'poetry' of a client's actions and words, as a way for the therapist to understand the client through the latter's own creativity (McNiff, 1998; Moon, 2003; Rogers, 1993; Rubin, 1999; Silverstone, 1993). Although criteria for aesthetic or 'high' art will not be activated (because they are not the aim) the client's processes will be observed through both artistic and psychological lenses. The use of multi-modal shifts may also be activated to enhance creativity.

Overall skills to practise

- *The elusive techniques of genuineness, creativity, authenticity, and acceptance of the other* are difficult to learn because they are so connected to inner character traits rather than to formal acquisition of knowledge. However, they need constant and evolving work to maintain. Silverstone suggests focusing on the inner critic and on roles such as persecutor, victim, and saviour, to find a 'neutral' inner stance (Silverstone, 1993).

- *Knowledge of art materials and methods* and the ability to create an art studio setting that enable the client to focus on creativity and supports those who are stuck (Moon, 2003).
- *The development of inner creativity or an 'artist identity'* through constant self-art is based on the assumption that one cannot encourage creativity in others without developing creativity of the self as an ongoing discipline. This might include keeping a sketchbook, going to exhibitions, doing an art class, and creating an art space at home (Allen, 1995).
- *The ability to observe the client through creative aesthetic lenses* enables the aesthetic distance with which to understand the client in a non-judgemental way. This can be practised (Moon, 2003; Robbins, 1999).

Art-based skills to practise

- Explore different types of art materials, and enable yourself to create whatever you feel needs to be expressed right now.
- Write down thoughts about the image, and then continue to do more art making on the issue, alternating between art making and art observing.
- Create a 'studio space' in your life that enables you to engage with art in an ongoing way.
- Use intentionality to define an issue you are concerned with right now, and then create art around the issue, using insights from the art to reframe and think about the issue. Continue this process until you feel you have resolved the issue.
- Use aesthetic distance to write a poem or draw a picture of a client you are concerned about.
- Explore the roles of rescuer, persecutor, and victim in your life.
- Create images of inner critics and conduct a dialogue with them.
- Create images of the people who have been 'humanistic' role models who helped you in your life. Think how to emulate them.

Chapter 6

Art as experience
Art therapy and gestalt

The contribution of this theory to art therapy is central in that it is based on spatial and sensual rather than verbal concepts. It also leans on art's major role as being communicative with others, and with self. The focus, first on emotional experience, and second on organizing this into a cognition and reorganization of parts and whole, are inherent to art therapy and to expressive therapy, creating an intense and interactive art therapy methodology.

Gestalt focuses on the experiential side of humanist theories, namely the importance of experiencing past and present feelings. Gestalt is also concerned with the integration of the different needs of the individual within the interactive contexts of his or her life. This holistic life picture – shifting needs in the different areas of spiritual, relational, physical, cognitive, and social elements that all interact with each other and with past experiences – is the overall gestalt of one's life. Fritz Perls, founder of this theory, and trained in psychoanalysis, describes reality as a continuing shift of overall context, and thus the 'gestalt'; in other words, the whole, at any given time, is made of a set of dominant and background needs. This enables an evolving relationship between past and present, and between different areas of the self. The self emerges as dynamic, multifaceted, and constantly evolving. The subject – is the immediate needs, while the "background", is the overall context of one's life. By becoming part of the gestalt, meaning is created through looking at the overall patterns of the gestalt of one's life, as new needs or themes constantly emerge and old ones recede. People can adopt false and avoidant selves, until they connect with their emotions (Bar-Yoseph, 2012; Belgrad, 1998; Perls, 1992).

The problem is therefore a lack of ability to reintegrate the past or present conflict into the overall gestalt of one's life at any given time. The solution is to experience one's emotions (rather than only to reach intellectual understanding of one's problems – past and present) within the body in the present moment, witnessed by others, and from this to reach an intellectual reintegration of different parts of the self, or different needs.

The social context of this theory can be seen in the influence of Perl's training as a psychoanalyst on his focus on experiencing repressed feelings. It can also be understood as the focus on the importance of authentic emotional connection over intellectual understanding within the counter-culture that was in opposition to the objectivist and behaviourist trust of psychology in the USA at the time (Belgrad, 1998; Leary, 1994; Sokal, 1984).

As a macro application of the theory, gestalt is often practised in a group context, where the group learns from an individual's experience and takes part in its enactment and expression. Because a person comprises many different facets of self, individuals can identify with different parts of others, thus forming a group identity. Directions such as drama therapy, and encounter groups that also focus on intense experiencing of emotions, often use gestalt methods (Greenberg, 2002).

Communities as well as individuals need to explore the different components of their overall gestalt, as well as experience things that preventing them from moving onwards. This may include community traumas and developing needs, that can be enacted and reintegrated into the overall backdrop of the community and its present needs, as in playback theatre (Huss, 2012a, 2013; Waller, 1993).

The role of art in gestalt concepts is essential because the stress is on experiencing and expressing emotions, and on utilizing the senses; art becomes a space that bridges emotion and cognition – therefore a central methodology. The concept of a gestalt, that is, an integrative and multifaceted identifty comprised of interacting parts, is by definition visual, and spatial. Gestalt's focus on others witnessing one's emotions leans to the performance and communicative element of art. The concept of art as a multi-model and interactive whole is at the basis of the multi-model theories of expressive therapy (Rhyne, 1991; Robbins, 1994; Rogers, 2007; Silverstone, 1993).

Within the 'core conditions' of the humanistic setting, the therapist works actively to create an evolving and interactive gestalt of the client's lifelong background problems. This involves the therapist searching for words to describe the emotions, and for connections between body and emotion (e.g. 'show me where you feel this emotion'). Another more analytical element is the testing of the relationship between the whole gestalt and the current problem. The therapist is directive and able to initiate multi-model activities that integrate the message.

The therapy evaluation is based on the developing ability of the client to express and feel her feelings in the here and now, and as a result, on how well she manages to create new integrations of parts of herself and of her current concerns into the overall gestalt of her life.

Visual evaluation will include the intensifying experiential and sensual elements of art expressions as process rather than as product (Rhyne, 1991). Evaluation can also include complexity, flexibility, and integration of the art works as they become more whole gestalts that encompass different parts of the self.

Supervision includes the humanistic attention to relationship as well as thinking about how to creatively guide the client into expressing and thus feeling emotions in the present art therapy sessions. Another direction might be for the supervisor to help the therapist to understand the relationship between the parts and the whole in the client's overall gestalt. This can occur through art work.

Research could include descriptive case studies, methodologies for enhancing emotional connection, and exploration of the visual relationships between parts and whole, and background and object in clients' art work.

As in all humanistic viewpoints, a critique of this theory is the lack of social and intercultural context from the perspective of social theories. In terms of dynamic theories, the focus on externalized and dramatic manifestations of emotion may be a superficial solution. Furthermore, the danger of experiencing intense emotions for people who have strong defences are not addressed in this theory. And same applies to people who have undergone traumatic experiences (Sokal, 1984).

Central concepts exemplified through case study

Layers of neurosis

The phony or false level of self is resistant to real interaction with others or the environment, which includes the empty or avoidant self and the overwhelming nature of emotions when they are experienced. These stages have to be got through to reach the true experience of self in the present.

> When Sharon (C3) first drew her shapes, she expressed her phony and avoidant self. When Rina (B2, B3) split her experience, she was also expressing her neuroses and avoidant self.

Experiencing things in the here and now

In light of the above, the overall aim therefore is to experience emotions in the present, rather than only to understand the past cognitively, as in dynamic therapy. The ability of art to create sensual arousal is an important method for experiencing feelings in the present.

> When Shoshana drew her red and black circle in oil pastels, expressing her anger (D2) she engaged her body in intense drawing and she had tears in her eyes. The image was not analysed, but finding words for her emotions were encouraged. Shoshana was asked to express herself as the black contour of the circle and then as the red centre of the circle, and to let the red centre talk to her original white spot (D1).
>
> Rina (B 1, 2, 3) was asked to show in movement how her body felt when in the black side of her picture, and how it felt in the colourful side.

Figure and ground

These concepts can be directly translated to spatial and colour relations where techniques such as collage enable us to explore the interrelations between the parts and the whole by focusing sometimes on parts of a composition and sometimes on the whole.

Avital (D3) then integrated her 'figure' of intense anger into the 'background' of the circles of others, into an overall gestalt of survivors of abuse as flower shapes.

Rina (B4) also integrated both black and white sides of her dissociation into a single gestalt of a mandala, which contained them both as an integrative possibility.

Interaction with others

In order to interact genuinely, internal and emotional parts of self must be shared and accepted by others.

Shoshana (A) expressed her fear about medical invasion of fertility treatments, and this fear was validated and accepted by the group. After that, she could move on to accepting the fear. Avital (D1) expressed her sense of self as nothingness, and this experience was validated, enabling her to move on.

Working the theory: art therapy skills and techniques

Visual techniques

Setting

The setting should include a room with art materials, dramatic props, and maybe musical instruments; this array of art materials is to encourage interaction. Art materials may be chosen according to their sensual impact, and gestalts will be created through integrative techniques such as collage and the use of multi-model shifts between the senses (McNiff, 1998; Robbins, 1999. There is often room for a group context.

Art processes

The art therapist aims to be creative and interactive, often directly initiating art activities that are built to connect to the most intense emotions, utilizing art expression to intensify and embody any emotional issue that arises. Art processes are directed by the therapist, aiming to create intense sensory and expressive situations; the art therapist will actively encourage full creative articulation and space for each of the client's different, and often opposing, emotions, as well as facilitate ways to integrate them. The art work is thus a constantly evolving process that does not become a final product.

The art therapist aims to constantly shift between the whole issue and the various parts of the gestalt that make up its composition. The therapist is able to 'enter' an art product experientially, rather than just analytically. This can include creating dialogue between parts of the product, or describing the emotions created by colours and shapes. For example, if a client describes his current problem as conflicts with his boss, and mentions his anger at his father for not keeping contact after divorce, the therapist may suggest depicting this anger, visually or dramatically, by 'talking' to the father and showing how this felt in the body. This feeling, once expressed, may be connected to problems in his present gestalt, with his boss, and maybe the role of anger in the overall collage of his life can be shifted in size and colour (McNiff, 1998; Robbins, 1999).

As in humanistic theory, the first stage of art analysis is to focus more on experiencing and catharsis, than on an intellectual unravelling. In the second stage, the art therapist and client can shift and reorganize the overall gestalt in visual terms. The analysis is thus based in changing the different parts of the overall gestalt (Johnson, 1999; Kapitan, 2003; McNiff, 1998; Moon, 2003; Rogers, 2007; Rhyne, 1991; Silverstone, 1993).

Overall skills to practise

- *The ability to create an experiential, sensory 'translation' of the problem through art materials,* art processes, and the use of the body to connect the client to his emotions through art.
- *This includes ability to shift between art modalities* in order to stay at the experiential level.
- *The therapist is able to actively connect between the client's specific issues and overall gestalt* through constant exploration and compositional reintegration of elements of self on a visual level. This means shifts to focusing on parts rather than focusing on the whole.
- *The therapist is able to 'enter' an art product experientially, rather than analytically.* This can include through dialoguing between parts of the product, or through describing the most and least comfortable part of the image, or the place in the body that different colours and shapes are experienced.
- *The ability to be directive, creative and confrontational* with clients about art products to enable this experiential level.

Art-based skills to practise

- Draw a conflict expressed as two different fish depicting the different sides of the conflict. Add them into a sea background that includes other areas of your life. Enact a conversation between the fish; other sea elements can also join in. Finally, create a solution that includes either choosing a single fish, or creating an integrated or new fish.
- Draw an issue that is a problem for you at present, create a collage of your present life and integrate the issue into the overall collage (shape or colour).
- Practise finding a voice, movement, and character for a painful emotion or experience from the past. Include other people as witnesses or as voices within the collage.

Chapter 7

Art as development
Art therapy and developmental theories

The contribution of developmental theory to art therapy is its direct connection between emotional-cognitive and social development, and art development. The focus on developmental stages over a lifetime also enables a model for working with different stages rather than only children. The theory has obvious contributions for psycho-educational work with children who missed out on school, or on emotional stages due to wars or disasters, or poverty and neglect of family or of country. As previously stated, art is shown as able to fill in gaps in cognitive and emotional developmental milestones. The concrete art product enables different overlapping developmental stages to be addressed simultaneously; and the emotional-cognitive element of art enables the clients to think of themselves as evolving and holistic people.

Developmental theory within humanistic theory conceives of people as constantly developing and evolving throughout life in the direction of self-fulfilment and self-actualization. For example, a girl who did not receive love and acceptance in childhood from her father (or mother) can find that love at a later stage from her partner. A child stuck at latency age due to learning difficulties, can return to study at a later stage, and succeed. Each developmental stage brings a new opportunity to correct former developmental stages and this process continues over the lifetime. This is in contrast to Freud's focus on early childhood conflicts as becoming calcified, which set the stage for rigid defences in later life (Freud, 1936). In accordance with the humanistic theories, this developmental standpoint is dynamic rather than static and is also holistically constructed from physical, emotional, and cognitive elements that are interactive with society as a whole (Erikson, 1993, 1998; Weems and Costa, 2005). The different challenges include constant integrations of emotional, cognitive, and social development. According to Erikson, these stages are universal and set, and each stage focuses around a specific dilemma between self versus society (see below for more details) (Erikson, 1993; Valsiner, 1997; Weems and Costa, 2005).

According to developmental theory, the problem is becoming trapped within a developmental stage that does not let the person continue evolving, or does not have the conditions to allow the person to successfully pass through a developmental stage.

The solution to the problem is to symbolically resole the developmental dilemma in order to continue to the next stage, and to face the challenges of the next stage more successfully.

The social context is the overall humanistic focus on the potential for self-actualization as an ongoing process. This focus merges with education and aims to develop the whole person rather than just to impart formal learning. As stated, the focus on childhood and on early education in childhood adopts art as a central method of enhancing as well as visually concretizing this overall emotional and cognitive development. Therefore, stages of children's drawing and expressive behaviour have been carefully studied (Belgrad, 1988; Gardner, 1993; Lowenfield, 1987).

Macro implications inform the assumption that life stages are universal and can create developmentally appropriate challenges for groups at the same stage. For example, a care home may be dealing with old people's acceptance of death but still building a satisfying life narrative. The culture or community as a whole can also be seen as undergoing different developmental stages and shifts, such as the honeymoon, reality, and working stages of groups (Yalom, 1994).

The role of art is especially suited to developmental theories because it concretely manifests, enacts and enhances developmental stages as shown in the finished art product (Di Leo, 1973; Goodnow, 1977[1926]; Horowitz, 2009; Kellogg, 1993) but also in the interactive processes of art making (Malchiodi, 1997; Williams and Wood, 1987). Art encourages physical, motor, cognitive, and emotional development (Gardner, 1993; Matthews, 1994).

The art therapist's role is to actively guide, mediate, and encourage the cognitive-emotional and social processes appropriate to each developmental stage as well as to identify and address conflicts in relation to prior stages directed, or open art interventions.

Evaluation will be according to developmental art manifestations that point to the cognitive and emotional level of maturity of the drawer. Regressions in cognitive levels can be understood as developmental delays or as emotional regression (Di Leo, 1973; Goodnow; 1977[1926]). The overall interaction and social behaviour of the client with the therapist and materials is another zone to evaluate development (Malchiodi, 1998b; Rubin, 1999).

Supervision will focus on the different developmental stages, both present and past, which emerge in the client's art work, and on ways to encourage further development using the art process, materials, and type of product created.

Research will be a focused case study, using a developmental meta-theory for analysis. Research can also explore the overall interaction between techniques and specific developmental stages (Rubin, 1999; Williams and Wood, 1987).

Another direction will be to explore the manifestation of different universal and culturally specific developmental stages within the context and compositional elements of art (Horowitz, 2009; Huss et al., 2012a; Kellogg, 1993; Kroup, 1995).

One can critique this theory because it defines a rigid sequence of universal developmental milestones that do not take into account culture, class, ethnicity, gender, or overall difference. For example, collective cultures put less stress on individuation and more on adherence to the collective values, and so developmental milestones are defined differently (Dwairy, 2004; Sue, 1996; Viney and King, 1998). This diversity is also expressed in children's art. For instance, most African children are not used to translating depth perception into image and cannot generally draw perspective, while children from Arab cultures draw more decoratively than realistically in accordance with their culture's visual aesthetic. Chinese children focus on realistic drawing from a very early age, which is considered developmentally inappropriate in Western society (Allen, 1988; Burman, 2007; Elkins, 2008; Hudson, 1960; Viney and King, 1988). We can gather from this that art development emerges not as a universal but as culturally contextualized.

Central stages of development as demonstrated through case study

Trust versus mistrust

This primary stage is concerned with the sense of trust in the world that the infant receives through a consistent and sensitive caretaker, who mediates pleasant interactions with the physical world and helps to deal with unpleasant ones.

The art therapist confirms, approves, and mirrors the child's first efforts to initiate marks on the page, encourages the evolving control of the child – who begins to see a connection between his markings and what is left on the page – and thus the child learns that the world is a safe, pleasant place through the therapist's accepting presence and through different positive experiences with the materials. This develops in parallel with words, and with overall symbolic self-expression.

> *Rina (C3) drew a girl according to a schema that reflects an earlier stage of development, the stage when she was abused. Her overall cognitive and emotional development was stopped by the traumatic experience and this is reflected in the composition of the drawn girl.*

Autonomy versus shame and doubt

The child gradually gains control of his physical needs and of his social behaviour, and becomes self-regulating, through many mistakes and 'meltdowns'. Lack of this ability at autonomy leaves him feeling worthless and shameful. In terms of art, the child learns to gradually control art materials and their outcome on the page. Emotions are sublimated and modulated through symbolic expression. The therapist is able to appreciate this effort, and help avoid or reframe situations of lack of control with art, by helping with materials, enabling free choice, and enabling a zone of autonomy and control.

> *Shoshana (A1) started with a black stain that was at a very regressed and primary level. In her next image (A2), she proceeded to a latency stage composition that organizes space and colours in logical rather than emotional or abstract concepts. Her next image (A3) climbed on to the next adolescent developmental stage: an abstract description of nature*

that contains emotions. And her final image of the baby inside the shapes (A4) was at an adult symbolic level. When given the core conditions of acceptance and authentication of her experience, she was able to 'grow' her emotional and cognitive developmental stages alone.

Initiative versus guilt

The aim of this stage is that the child feels he/she counts, and that he/she can communicate and initiate interactions effectively, rather than in an anti-social way. Visual schemas become more developed, stable, and complex. The child draws what is most important to him in terms of his most intense cognitive and emotional experiences, aiming to initiate their expression within symbolic form. The child thus becomes an active communicator with others, learning to listen as well as to talk. He/she becomes an active member of a group and can cooperate, for example, on a joint art initiative.

Industry versus inferiority

The developmental challenge within latency is to become a hard-working and successful member of a group but in a reality outside the family. Art becomes reality-oriented, with elements such as perspective, overall background, proportion, as central. The child will exhibit much industry to reach these results, and the ensuing praise for the art product.

> *Avital (D) in the beginning didn't draw at all, but then moved from guilt to initiative on her page and gradually started initiating images (D1, D2, D3).*

Identity versus role confusion and intimacy versus loneliness

Within the teenage years, the cognitive and emotional levels are more sophisticated and integrated: search for identity is conceptualized in abstract terms and in the context of the peer culture. The challenge for young adults is to create intimacy with a partner but also to develop as an individual, to find their place in work and love. Within art, this can be expressed by being able to share inner emotions with the therapist, while also maintaining a sense of self.

> *In Shoshana's (A1) and Sharon's (C1) first images, we see that shapes do not touch and colours do not merge. Over time, both created more merging interactions between colours and shapes, which reflected their broadening definition of self, enabling more intimacy with others in the group.*

Developing versus stagnation

Given that the individual has resolved previous stages, her challenge in midlife is to continue developing and expressing herself, rather than to stagnate into a lack of meaning and vitality. In terms of art, the empty page enables her to redefine identity and self, and to explore aspects of self that are not normally expressed

> *We see that both Shoshana (1) and Avital (4) in their art work explored ways to continue developing rather than stagnating – through having a baby and through engaging in community work.*

Ego integrity versus despair

Towards the end of life, the challenge is to feel at one with how life has developed, and to be satisfied with one's choices. Art becomes a place to reflect on this process.

> *Shoshana (D) had reached a stage of despair in midlife in that she defined her identity as invisible, a white dot. However, throughout her time with the group, she managed to overcome this despair and create meaning in her life by engaging with her pain and turning it into social action.*

Working the theory: art therapy skills and techniques

Verbal techniques

All types of reflection, interpretation, feedback and confrontation are suited to the perceived developmental needs of the client (Erikson, 1993). The therapist is also an active encourager or teacher of the skills needed in the current developmental stage, with a focus on behaviour as well as insight. The relationship is non-judgemental and enabling, but also directive and forward focused, aiming to encourage growth and helping to release former stages through developmentally appropriate skills and challenges (Heegaard, 2001; Magniant and Freeman, 2004; Masten, 2001; Stepney, 2001).

Visual techniques

Setting

The setting can be adjusted by choosing materials and directives specifically suited to the developmental needs of the client. For example, the controllability of materials in relation to motor development, and the ability of the materials to create a sensory experience for small children, a pleasing and gender-appropriate end product for latency children, or a youth culture appropriate medium such as video, or an abstract expressive directive for adolescents. A latency child can be offered pictures to copy, while a preschool child can be offered finger paints, and an older person with low motor control can be offered easily manipulated, but 'adult', materials. The art therapist adjusts and controls the setting to suit the overt and covert developmental needs of the client.

Art process

Art processes, therefore, offer developmentally appropriate art materials, directives (or not) and analyses of art work. The complexity is in combining the client's real and unresolved or regressed developmental stages. For example, for a latency-aged child, the therapist might be product-oriented and directive, but at the same time, might enable the use of wet and non-structured materials as part of the structured activity, such as colouring in a set of boxes with wet regressive paint, or creating a building, satisfying the need to explore early childhood issues of self-regulation, as well as creating a structured, reality-oriented product. Conversely, an adult in the intimacy versus individuation stage may be directed to work on different types of boundaries or contours between elements, exploring their intersection and permeability.

Art interpretation

According to the developmental stages, art interpretation is expressed in interactive art making as well as in the compositional and content characteristics of the product. The cognitive and emotional stages of the child are understood as combined within the art product, such as ability to symbolize, to notice detail, to express trust, and sense of a coherent environment. Overall, art's development is in the direction from less to more motor control, and from less to more ability to integrate detail and abstract concepts with increasingly complex symbolization. Development is characterized in shifts from emotional to cognitive focus at different times in life (Kellogg, 1993; Malchiodi, 1998b; Williams and Wood, 1987). Art can express the present developmental stage, according to some parameters such as context but also, according to other parameters in the same image, reveal the past stages in composition. For example the drawing of a family by a latency child might have detail and realistic proportions, except for the (problematic) father figure who has much less detail and less exactitude in the contours (Malchiodi, 1998b; Matthews, 1994; Rubin, 2001; Williams and Wood, 1987).

Overall skills to practise

- *Becoming familiar with developmental stages:* the cognitive-emotional and social needs of each stage.
- *Understanding manifestations of each developmental stage* and their manifestations in art content and composition.
- *Being able to actively create a social and art context* or directive that is suitable to the developmental stage of the client.
- *Working with developmental theory on dual interactive levels;* this includes understanding the client's current stage and past developmental stages that were not negotiated successfully, and working on both through art directives, materials, and processes.

Art-based skills to practise

- Create an image of the most meaningful and difficult stage of your life; and then understand it in terms of the above theory. What helped you develop and what is still stuck?
- Draw a linear narrative of your life giving each stage a symbol.
- Draw your present developmental stage and former stages as an interactive collage.
- Draw an image of your present life, using the compositional techniques typical of the most difficult stage of your life. Explore the relationship between content and composition.
- Note the current but also covert developmental stages of people you interact with, and try to address both levels.

Chapter 8

Art as telling and retelling

Art therapy and narrative theory

Narrative theories' contribution to art therapy is that they focus on the ability of art to give transformative form and meaning to experience and to communicate it to the self and to others. While narrative therapy is usually associated with words, within our media-infused society today, personal and cultural narratives are often focused on images as well as words. Art therapy itself uses images to generate new words, and expands words with images; thus there is an intense potential connection between art therapy and narrative therapy.

Narratives enable us a symbolic space to organize, contain, and therefore control the endless stimuli and challenges of our experience. Communicating our experience to others through stories is the natural way to gain feedback and fresh interpretations and comments from others and from ourselves, which facilitate shifts to more enabling meanings attributed to the stories. Narrative theory continues the humanistic focus on how a person experiences or interprets what happens. This phenomenological and subjective interpretation of life's events, when positive, is what creates meaning in life and what leads to more enabling actions and better events. Thus, our lives are witnessed and confirmed. Narrative theory explores not only what is told, but also how things are told (Epston, 1996; Payne, 2006; White, 2007).

One problem according to this theory is when we can't tell our story because we don't have an enabling audience, or due to lack of coherence, trauma, or negative connotations that would allow us to find a positive frame for the story.

A solution is to find those to whom we can communicate our story; who provide core conditions of acceptance and new insights or perspectives of the story. The aim is to find a symbolic container within which to reframe meanings of the narrative so as to create a more enabling explanation of the painful events of our lives (Frankl, 1985; Save and Nuutinen, 2003; Sclater, 2003).

The social context of this theory is the humanistic and existential focus on the subjective self as being able to generate meaning and to shift meaning. Constructivist theories also focus on how people understand, and from their understanding construct reality. This evolved to a focus on more positive meanings in the context of positive psychology orientations, outlined in Chapter 9 (Besley, 2002).

A macro application of this theory is that communities as well as individuals need to tell and to retell their collective narrative in order to incorporate changes effectively. Reinterpretation of traditional narratives can preserve the tension between community homeostasis and change. Community narratives become a container for group traumas and enable peacemaking with the past and point the way to coping in the future (Darley and Heath, 2008; Davis and Sheridan, 2010; Frankl, 1985; Save and Nuutinen, 2003; Sclater, 2003). This chapter will outline how a group may be empowered by sharing the same reality, which creates a joint narrative by incorporating the shared impact of social circumstances on their personal lives.

The role of art in narratives may be both visual and verbal, and may be made up of both content and form, and of the relationship between content and form. Often narratives have visual and verbal components, especially within media-infused culture that tells its stories through images alternated with words, as in Facebook, comics, PhotoVoice, and others. These connect to art therapy because of the role attributed to the visual, creative, and symbolic telling of stories using metaphors, symbols, and different tensions between content and composition.

The role of the art therapist is to encourage the client to use verbal and visual methods to tell his story and to help reframe or transform the existing narrative to the most psychologically enabling form through art and words. This means that both client and therapist actively engage in the creation of the narrative on the level of what and how, or on the level of content and composition. Both focus on the art product rather than on the relationship. Beyond analyses of the narrative, the aim is to enhance understanding, acceptance, meaning, and agency through the narrative in order to create new and more enabling perspectives on the content of the narrative, or on the self as expressed in the narrative. This can be done through additional art work, or additional interpretations of existing art work (Liebmann, 1996; Moon, 2008; Pizaro, 2004; Riley, 1997; Sclater, 2003).

Traumatic experiences are encoded non-verbally into the mind; by creating a visual narrative of experience, these elements can be raised, and reinterpreted with the verbal mind, enabling their integration and reframing (Hass-Cohen, 2003; Kaye and Bleep, 1997; Malchiodi, 2012; Warren, 2008). This can include actively suggested changes in the image's process of creation, and in relation to the meanings that it elicits when observed: reframing, reinterpretation, and confrontation of elements in the content and in the composition of the image. The therapist may suggest and use visual techniques that incorporate existing images such as photos, as well as constructing images, using multi-model methods of eliciting new narratives from existing ones. The products can be kept private, or shared with particular people or the general public, depending on the client's decision and feelings.

Evaluation of the therapy will focus on how the narrative is developing and changing in the direction of a more enabling narrative that is therapeutic for the client. Visual evaluation will explore the evolving contents of the image as well as shifts that the client tells about his images in the narrative, in terms of their ability to enable new perspectives.

Supervision will focus on the interaction of the client and therapist within the creating of the narratives, as well as on the content and compositional elements of how the narrative has developed and how to expand its therapeutic potential. It is as if client and therapist gaze at but also construct the narrative together, and then supervisor and therapist analyse this process and content of construction. The focus is on the narrative rather than the relationship.

Research can be based on case studies that explore the methodology of creating and shifting narratives: case studies that tell the narrative – or the end product, or the narrative – as a story or art work in itself. Narrative therapy is closely connected to narrative research methods. Indeed, Sclater (2003) claims that telling one's story as a research participant is in itself therapeutic.

Qualitative narrative research is a developing field. Of late there has been an explosion in art-based narrative methods, as shown in the rise in art-based research, visual culture, visual anthropology, social art, and the art therapies within the social sciences (Eisner, 1997; Emmison and Smith, 2000; Huss, 2011, 2012b; Lawler, 2002). Qualitative narrative research includes analysing existing images in media, creating images, and using PhotoVoice. Analysis might focus on the content of the visual or verbal narrative. This could be in terms of its central themes; in terms of the relationship between content and composition; in terms of central symbols and compositional elements such as repetition; or in terms of an analysis of the narrative according to a grounded, social, or psychological theory. But it can also be focused, as in humanistic theories, on the narrator's own analysis of what she considers most important. Indeed, drawing an image and then talking about the image may be a way to intensify the interpretive voice of the research participant or client, who first defines the contents in his image, and second, explains the content. Interestingly, this direction is used less in art therapy, where the focus is on art measurement or analysis according to psychological meta-theories (Gilroy *et al.*, 2012; Huss, 2012a; Wadeson, 2002).

A critique of this theory could be that according to dynamic theory it does not work deeply enough to take into account defences against changing viewpoints and narratives. From a social perspective, it does not take into account reality and the impact of oppression, as it claims that changing the perspective of the narrative is enough (Bronner, 2011; DeCarvalho, 1991; Skaif and Heil, 1988).

Central concepts illustrated in the case study

Working on a narrative can involve the following stages.

Starting with a problem-saturated narrative – verbal versus visual problems:

> *Shoshana (A 1) described her image as her wish to get pregnant but fear of the gyneacological tests that it involved. Her black centre was drawn but not verbalized; it is the centre of the narrative that could not yet be verbalized but that could be shown. The black centre as the sexual abuse is the reason for the problem in the narrative that is expressed visually.*

Continuing the effort to name or give a title to the problem and exploring its effect on the person is an external event rather than an inherent part of the person and contextualizing the problem within social reality.

The words Shoshana wrote on the image from a popular song about how bad the world is, while not her own, begin to be the solution through naming the problem. She reframed the sexual abuse or black square as not inside herself, but inside society. This is a reframing of the narrative defining the problem as an external event.

Witnessing the story by people who understand and can help affirm and redefine it.

We see that the 'blackness' that the women drew in different ways became a way to witness each other's experience while also expanding upon it.

Narratives constitute a distanced place to confront painful content.

Sharon (C4) explained that the hands in her image were helping her, and this interpretation was confronted by the group looking at the image, who stated that the hands were not helping her as they did not touch her although she was bleeding. This difficult confrontation with Sharon's denial of the abuse could take place in the distanced and symbolic conversation about the image, rather than directly about Sharon.

Constructing one's story is a therapeutic event in itself: the act of organizing an experience into a symbolic and narrative form, creating a coherent whole, with levels of symbolization, organization, and meaning enable a sense of control over the problem leading to dialogue about its content, in a distanced and contained form. This in itself can be considered therapeutic and enables ownership of the problem (Huss, 2009a).

Narratives are dynamic and evolving constructs through interaction of observer and creator: in keeping with the humanistic stance, the narratives here are recounted (to self and others) and their meanings are constantly reconstructed, negotiated, and evolved.

We saw that Shoshana shifted between different versions of the image of the black centre until it became a womb with a baby inside. This enabled her to reconstruct her story through the different compositions of her image. The women's comments that legitimized her fear of medical intervention to have a baby also verbally reframed the issue.

Working the theory: art therapy skills and techniques

Verbal techniques

Verbal techniques include active listening, reflecting, and feedback. However, active reframing, interpreting, and confrontation of contents to create a more psychologically enabling narrative are done within the zone of the narrative rather than in the zone of the client's direct reality. The shift of the therapeutic content to the narrative rather than talking about direct reality is more distanced and enables fewer defences; while the power of witnessing, owning, and sharing a narrative is therapeutic in its own right (Jones, 2003; Moon, 2008; Riley, 1993, 1997; Riley and Malchiodi, 1994).

Images may be understood as creating a broader and looser metaphorical space then a verbal narrative and as such are open to more interpretations. In other words, speaking around an image will shift the discourse of the narrative to visual elements, enabling visual insights, creating more emotive, personal, and expressive formulations than words, which are often calcified into set issues. Narrative therapy and art therapy have in common that they focus on the relationship between content and composition, understanding meaning to be at the meeting place between them. Both utilize an analysis of compositional elements and may include verbal and visual metaphors, symbols, repetitions, space division, voice, intensity, velocity, and additional elements taken from both art and literature.

Settings

The setting will encourage art use to create visual narratives, enabling a choice of materials that create different associations, and symbolic messages to enrich the narrative. The setting may include ready-made elements for faster illustrative narrative forms, and classic art materials for more process-oriented embodied forms (Schaverien, 1999).

Art process

Within a narrative about something painful from the past (e.g. giving up a child to social services) the therapist can verbally reframe that this was a brave thing to do, as a way to help the child. The pain but also love for the child may be depicted in the form of symbol or colour in an image, and these feelings can be accessed through the image. Narrative theories have different ways to work with a narrative in a structured model, such as starting with a problem-saturated narrative, giving a title to the problem, exploring its effect on the narrator, and contextualizing it within a social reality.

Art interpretation

As in humanistic theories, the analysis is ongoing, flexible, and collaborative and not based on a meta-theory. Rather it is based on collaborative analysis of the relationship between content and form in both visual and verbal elements, and then the relationship between verbal and visual elements, by therapist and client together. The aim is to reach a more psychologically enabling narrative (Payne, 2006; White, 2007).

Overall skills to practise

- *Learning to listen to the 'composition' of verbal narratives* that include metaphors, symbols, texts amounts, repetitions, themes, and linear organization of ideas over time, and to apply these to visual compositions as well.
- *Learning to actively reframe ideas through the narrative* to suggest changes that reframe the content – through suggesting additional art work, or additional words.
- *Learning to elicit multiple and changing narratives* about images through different techniques, such as the cognitive, analytical, phenomenological and immersion techniques as ways to talk about a picture, outlined in the earlier chapters.
- *Shifting from art to words and from expression to interpretation* as part of an ongoing dialectical process.

Art-based skills to practise

- Create a story with images and words, about a central event in your life that concerns you at present.
- Develop the visual part only and then the verbal part only.
- Compare visual and verbal parts in terms of what you learnt from each.
- Create a visual narrative about something that concerns you at present from multiple perspectives, multiple materials, or multiple symbols.

Chapter 9

Art as the positive

Art therapy and positive psychology

The contribution of positive theories to art therapy is in their potential to connect to art as a concrete zone for envisaging solutions. Although CBT has not been much developed in art therapy literature, it too has the potential to connect with art as a concrete zone of action, as a self-regulative activity, and as an actual way of confronting negative thoughts. Art becomes a zone in which to affirm, envisage, define, prioritize, and change reality. It is a visual confrontation with unconscious perceptions (rather than unconscious conflicts). This shifts art therapy from an irrational exploration of the emotional to a visual tool to organize, control, and define issues. Interestingly, the neurological findings paradoxically return us to dynamic theories where art is considered a preverbal or preconscious type of encasement of experience (Freud, 1900; Hass-Cohen, 2003).

Cognitive behavioural therapy aims to shift negative perceptions of self, and of one's actions, into more positive ones. On the one hand, this is a continuation of the narrative focus on positive reframing of experience; and on the other, it is based in behavioural theories that highlight how perceptions can change behaviour and how positive experiences can change perceptions (Bandura, 1977; Dryden and Neenan, 2004; Elkins, 2008; Huss *et al.*, 2010; Skinner, 1988).

The focus is on behaviourally training the mind to shift to positive perceptions of self and other issues. This follows the connection between mind and body, developed in neuroscience. Mind-body theories developed the concept of the person as a physiological whole, whose mind, body, emotions, and behaviours are in fact neurological functions that can be changed through altering the chemistry of the brain. The development of neurological science shows that both traumatic experiences and positive relationships physically affect and change the brain. Therefore, art as impacting on experiences, emotions, and physical self-regulating can alter the neurology of the brain. The connection between emotion, thought, and physical symptoms, mediated by neurons and different brain areas, became the 'science' of the soul (Abraham, 2001; Bryant *et al.*, 2003; Perry *et al.*, 1995; Van der Kolk *et al.*, 2001; Wills, 2008).

Theories of positive psychology also assume that there is always stress, but the interesting question is how people deal with stress; in other words, what creates resilience (Antonovsky, 1979; Hobfoll, 2001; Masten, 2001). Perceptions of meaning, management, comprehension (sense of coherence), together with self-regulatory physical behaviours and medication (if needed) all work together to cope effectively with stress. This is based not on diagnosing pathology, but on understanding how people cope, what people do that works, or that enhances resilience in stressful situations (Antonovsky, 1979; Masten, 2001; Saleeby, 1996).

The problem is therefore not the negative things that happen to us, but the negative perceptions or cognitions that we develop around them. This develops into stress, and ensuing negative mind sets, which may lead to negative lifestyles. The problem is thus not defined as based in the past, or as a lack of authentic self or core conditions, or unjust society, but rather as based in the mind, and in behaviour, in terms of how we perceive all of these elements.

The solution is to train oneself to discard negative thought patterns and to focus on positive cognitions, behaviours, and recourses. This focus can be practised and learnt through a combination of physical cognitive and emotional skills: attention to diet; relaxation; self-regulation and medication, if needed; mindfulness that focuses on now rather than on the past; avoidance of stress; and systematically training the brain to avoid negative mind sets. Spirituality as an uplifting, reframing and self-regulating technique may also be used.

The extension of behaviourist theories shows that not only what one does, but also how one thinks about what one does, will influence behaviour in the future. Neurological developments point to the connection between brain and emotion, and between physical and emotional states. Another social influence is the postmodern conception of identity that deconstructs that of a coherent inherent 'self' that has to be analysed, or actualized, or find meaning, as in dynamic and humanistic theories. The postmodern self is constantly evolving and made up of mind, body, and spirit, which are in multifaceted interaction and thus can all be addressed in therapy. Another contextual element is the rise of neo-capitalism and the decline of the welfare state, which means that people and health systems cannot afford long-term interventions. The focus on 'evidence' of things working justifies the cost of the therapy, with a focus on what can be proven to work quickly (Gerken, 2001; Martin and Sugarman, 2000).

Macro applications can include enhancing positive narratives of a community, focusing on community resources rather than pathology, and on teaching self-regulation and prevention through enhancing positive behaviours and healthy lifestyles.

The role of art in biological and cognitive theories is the neurological and perceptual process, which occurs in visual data stored in the mind as a type of preverbal coding of experience – the most primary way of processing experience. Thus, accessing and then changing images – as in guided imagery, a central technique in CBT – is a first step to adjusting perceptions and thoughts, which are secondary to images. This can include creating positive images and using visualization of wished-for future outcomes as a way to influence behaviour and understanding on a primary level. Art can thus change perceptions of the past, and of the future (Jones, 2005; Kaye and Bleep, 1997; Malchiodi, 2012; Warren, 2008).

Art may also be analysed in terms of the cognitions that its content assumes. It becomes a way to concretize understandings, perceptions or viewpoints, and over time can show shifts in them (Csikszentmihalyi, 1990; Rosal, 2001; Sarid and Huss, 2010).

On a more mind-body note, art expression may be understood as a holistic activity that creates connections between mind, body, and emotion in a way that enables the organism to regulate its physiological and emotional over- and under-excitation. This is expressed in theories of creative processes, such as art making, that enhances mindfulness through enabling a mind-set of 'flow' and deep concentration (Bell and Robbins, 2007; Cary and Rubin, 2006; Csikszentmihalyi, 1990; De Petrillo and Winner, 2005; Fontana, 1993; Hass-Cohen, 2003; Hass-Cohen and Carr, 2008; Monti *et al.*, 2006). Art making also integrates left and right brain functions, and as such creates new neurological pathways between emotional and cognitive areas of the brain. These pathways enable flexibility of thought, opposed to the rigid, repetitive, or fragmented thinking when under stress or after trauma (Arrington, 2001; Hass-Cohen, 2003; Malchiodi and Perry, 2008; Sarid and Huss, 2010; Tuhiwai-Smith, 1999). Cognitively, creativity facilitates new perspectives and thus problem solving (Hass-Cohen, 2003; Kaye and Bleep, 1997; Malchiodi, 2012; Warren, 2008).

Evaluation is an ongoing part of the therapy, and clear measures of improvements in cognitions, behaviours, and self-regulation are monitored by the therapist and client, using charts, subjective evaluations (as in behaviourist theories), and observation of improvements in behaviour. The evaluation is the base for deciding on the therapy goals in each session. Clear improvements in more positive cognitions, self-regulation of mood, and overall coping aim to measure and monitor these developments, with joint responsibility for charting and monitoring specific predetermined improvements. Art can be used to monitor shifts in cognitions and in self-regulation (Hass-Cohen, 2003; Rosal, 2001).

Supervision will focus on skills to teach the client: the supervisor is more like a teacher and coach than an emotional container or analyser of processes and relationships. The focus is on techniques and on the evaluative process. As before, art works and art interventions are considered in terms of how they can help promote the desired cognitions and behaviours (Malchiodi and Perry, 2008; Malchiodi and Riley, 1996).

Research as evaluation is inherent to the overall therapy, as a method of empirically measuring the predefined outcomes. It is built into the intervention in that the process and results of the therapy are constantly monitored through questionnaires, checklists, homework, and discussions, as well as through observation of social and physical outcomes. The types of goals are clear and concrete, and thus easy to measure. This creates an 'evidence-based' definition of therapy that only continues if it is effective, and for as long as it is effective. The therapy provides the data for analysis (Byrant *et al.*, 2003; Cooper, 2008).

Much art therapy research has aimed to prove that art enables neurological emotional and self-regulation. Less research has focused on art and positive psychology and on transforming standpoints (Bell and Robbins, 2007; Curl, 2008; Gilroy, 2006; Mohanty, 2003).

A critique of this theory is that it may be too simplistic to assume that positive behaviours can be 'taught' regardless of complex defences. Its evaluation shows short-term improvement but often the measurement is not over the long term. As in Chapter 8, another criticism could be that this stance helps to perpetuate oppressive social realities because problems are defined as faulty cognitions, which defines failure as the client's problem rather than society's or the therapist's problem. The focus on simplistic outcomes, and on short-term therapy results, is another critique, attributed to the social context of neo-capitalism that aims to reduce care in health funds, which standardize to the lowest common denominator (Alcock, 1997; Foucault, 2000; Gerken, 2001; Jameson, 1991). Similarly, while it is helpful to prove art therapy's ability to change mood, this in effect reduces art to a type of 'pill', greatly reducing the potential richness of hermeneutic and creative processes that aim to touch and give form to man people's suffering, rather than only to eliminate it on the immediate level.

The role of the art therapist is to use art to regulate and calm over-excitation; stimulate depressed or under-excited symptoms; use art to access positive perceptions; and to concretize and visualize recourses and positive outcomes. Art can also be used to capture negative perceptions.

Central concepts exemplified through case study

Art as a self-regulating activity, through creating an experience of flow and mindful engagement that calms the system

> *The women (ABCD) all shifted from more rigid dissociated shapes in felt-tip pens, or not drawing at all, to gradually more complex, engaged and longer integrative art experiences, where they could reach an experience of immersion and flow in their continuing art works. They spent longer making art than at the beginning. This calm setting enabled them to address the difficult contents.*

Art as a preverbal codifying of disturbing experiences

Often traumatic images are coded in the more primal visual parts of the brain, because the mind cannot make sense of the experience due to its painful or meaning-shattering quality. Accessing these images, and transforming them, is a first step to verbally processing the experience.

> *Sharon (C2) did not 'see' the blood stain on the girl's skirt until her friends in the group pointed it out. This enabled her to access the traumatic experience and to reframe it according to reality, deciding that the hands in the picture were not 'helping' but rather disturbing her.*

Art connects between right and left brain functions, enabling connections between emotions and cognitions

This is important for processing experience in an ultimate way.

> *Avital (D3) started drawing a black circle and then realized it was anger and managed to connect to the emotion. Rina realized that her images were split along the middle, and understood that this paralleled her extreme black or white thinking.*

Art as concretizing solutions to problems and visualizing possible positive outcomes

Art may be problem solving, by providing manageability, comprehension, and meaning, as in the salutogenic theory (Antonovsky, 1979). Art may be shifting perceptions and visualizing solutions.

> *Shoshana (A4) drew a baby in her stomach as a visualization of where she wanted to reach, which enabled a sense of manageability towards the medical interventions she was scared of.*
>
> *Avital (D3) saw a possibility of uniting the images into a poster, and utilized her connections and resources to develop a social activist career out of her experience that created meaning.*
>
> *Rina created integrations on the page, which she then tried to create in her life by leaving her high-risk job and boyfriend (B3, B4). Sharon struggled to create images of a more authentic and integrated self (C3, C4). The images enabled both of them to reach more comprehension of their defences.*
>
> *The women started solving these issues through art which provided alternative visualizations of possible experiences, and in this way shifted real behaviours. The art created a sense of manageability and comprehension, and enabled them to explore fields of meaning, and of recourses.*

Working the theory: art therapy skills and techniques

Verbal techniques

The therapist actively teaches the client how to follow negative thoughts and to correct them, how to focus on strengths and positive solutions, and how to regulate the physical reactions to stress. These are all taught and practised in therapy and using behavioural homework for the client to internalize new thoughts and behaviour patterns and learn methods to self-regulate stress and to actively relax. The therapist is solution-focused, teaching the client so that he/she or she can internalize the theories and manage them themselves. This may include suggestions for healthy eating, calming practices, physical therapies, and exercises that emphasize the connection between mind and body, such as massage and yoga, and mindfulness.

Visual techniques

Setting

CBT, positive psychology, and mind-body settings focus on the self-directed and regulative potential of art making. This demands a calm setting, and art activities that enhance a positive sensory experience, such as filling in mandalas, and using water colours. CBT and positive psychology uses art as a way to concretize negative perceptions hidden in the composition, to illustrate thought processes, and to envisage solutions. Art materials can be more linear and minimal in terms of their sensory scope, enabling the client to illustrate ideas.

Art processes

According to this model, the therapist is directive and in charge of the art, which is a method to reach a predetermined aim. The therapist's aim is to use art to illustrate and concretize the problem, but also to focus on envisaging new solutions, shifting negative standpoints, and future goals. The creativity and strengths of the client are utilized: this may include, for example, a map of resources, a map of guiding values, and an image of where she want to be in a year, or a negative thought process that is transformed visually into a positive. In terms of using art to self-regulate the client, the focus is on the process: the art therapist may suggest using calming art materials, drawing mandalas, or creating images that utilize the holistic mind-body and flow component of art making to regulate the body, and to encourage mindfulness. It can include drawing an image of a safe space for stressful situations (Bell and Robbins, 2007; Csikszentmihalyi, 1990; Curl, 2008; De Petrillo and Winner, 2005; Hass-Cohen, 2003; Hass-Cohen and Carr, 2008; Henderson *et al.*, 2007; Huss and Sarid, 2011; Rosal, 2001; Warren, 2008; Zammit, 2001).

Art interpretation

Art interpretation is based on the outcome of the art (such as enhancing levels of self-regulation or stress reduction) or on the perceptions expressed in the art (such as negative perceptions in composition or content) or on the level of cognitive and behavioural shifts that the art enabled (such as positive visualizations of the future). Thus, the art is a method rather than a relevant product in its own right.

Overall skills to practise

- *Identifying negative perceptions in art composition and content* with the client and discussing ways to shift the image to a positive cognition that changes them (see below).
- *Exploring techniques and materials that calm the client* dealing with trauma or anxiety and help him to feel calm and self-regulated such as safe place drawings, use of mandalas, guided imagery.
- *Creating images of resources in day-to-day life.*

- *Visualizing positive outcomes to problems* and drawing the outcomes.
- *Addressing physical and emotional pain through creating images of healing colours* and shapes that reduce it.

Art-based skills to practise

- Envisage and draw a place that makes you feel safe and calm, commit it to memory, and try to enter and leave it in your mind over the day. Hang it up close to you so that you have time to internalize it.
- Draw a situation that created much stress for you and write down the situation. Try to access the perceptions and stress reactions through the composition and content of the image and write them down.
- Now shift the image with additional colours or other changes, to include your coping resources. Also, try and create a more positive interpretation of the situation using compositional elements and symbols to transform the image.
- Write down the reframing and the resources.
- Use the above technique with a sketchbook at work when feeling stressed, draw the problem, and also the solution.
- When flooded with feelings and thoughts, create a map, diagram, or visual list of the elements and organize them into a coherent composition. Translate this into a set of ways to address the problem.

Table 9.1 Humanistic theories: content, composition, and role of therapist

	Content	*Process*	*Therapist*
Humanistic	Helps explore authentic self	Preconscious and accessible	Enables client to undergo art processes and to translate them into meaning
Gestalt	Helps reorganize cognitions	Helps connect to emotions	Actively connects between art process and emotions and then cognitions
Developmental	Real stage of development	Process and composition, as stuck or emotional stage of development	Encourages developmental milestones in stuck and chronological stages of development
Narrative	The primary form of the narrative	Space to shift meanings in the narrative in content and composition	Encourages reframing an enabling narrative
CBT and mind-body	Shows perceptions Shows potential shifts	Enables shifts, emotional regulation, and cognitive perception	Teaches client to shift to positive perceptions and self-regulatory behaviours to shift conscious standpoints

Table 9.2 outlines the shifts within the overall theory in terms of each sub-theory.

Summary of humanistic theories

We see that humanistic and positive psychology theories focus on the inherent uniqueness, individuality, and potential of each person; a potential that blossoms when the core conditions of acceptance, respect, and fulfilment of basic needs are met. Art is a place in which to explore this meaning and to reach one's authentic self; it can only be interpreted by the subjective phenomenological experience of the artist-client. Thus, creativity becomes an encompassing and individual process. Art becomes a zone to create meaning and to reframe meanings, in existential and narrative theories, to connect to one's experiences, and to integrate different facets of experience according to gestalt theories. And art is a place to symbolically express and strengthen developmental challenges over a lifetime according to developmental theories. Art therefore becomes a path not to the unconscious, but to the authentic self.

The focus is not just on the process and product but also on how the product is interpreted. The focus is therefore on the possibility of multiple interpretations rather than a single external meta-theory. The phenomenological experience of self and of life is accessed, expressed, shared, and reorganized through art. Not having the core conditions that enable this process of exploration of self may be problematic; the solution is to create those conditions through art engagement. Within mind-body, CBT, and positive psychology orientations, this direction is interpreted as an active cognitive focus on the positive, on what works. Its holistic nature is interpreted as the connection between mind, body and emotions, or soul. Therefore, medical intervention can regulate emotions, and conversely, intervention can regulate the body. A critique of the humanist stance is that while it talks about core conditions in terms of relationships, it does not seriously address the impact of systems of oppression and social context, which do not enable self-actualization. It provides the illusion that a person only has to want to evolve, and to express herself, and she will be able to; but this is only true for people with enough financial and cultural power to do so.

From a dynamic perspective, humanistic theories do not take seriously the defences that make reaching and actualizing the self very difficult for people who have underdone serious damage or trauma.

Table 9.2 Summary of humanistic art therapy

	Humanistic	Gestalt	Narrative	Developmental	CBT and mind-body
Setting	Non–directed and rich in materials and art techniques	Multi-model including props and musical instruments	Illustrative materials such as crayons, magazines and collage materials, and general art materials	An array of materials and techniques that are set out by therapist in conjunction with developmental aim	Materials that create pleasant and positive experiences of flow, and materials that enable illustration and organization of concepts
Art process	Directed by client in the art room	Suggested by therapist to zoom in on an emotion with shifts between modules	Therapist and client work on creating visual and verbal narratives together	Therapist encourages client to undergo a specific developmentally appropriate directed art intervention	Directed by therapist to elicit a specific experience or to illustrate a specific concept
Art product	Is understood by client and is often reacted to with more art as an ongoing process of creation and of self-discovery	It is witnessed by therapist. Often the group and others can intervene within the art product to give it additional focus and meanings	The art product is worked on carefully to contain all of the meanings reached in its making; it is often reacted to with more narratives	Art product is less important than process; it is measured in terms of developmental level	Art product is less important than the experiences or cognitions that enable
Therapist's role	To encourage engagement of client with the art and create core conditions for this	To intensify the communicative and sensory emotional experience of the art	To collaboratively build the narrative and to witness it	To encourage developmentally appropriate growth through art processes	To direct, teach, and focus the art to reach new cognitions and new experiences

Table 9.2 (cont.)

	Humanistic	Gestalt	Narrative	Developmental	CBT and mind-body
Art evaluation	Is evaluated by the therapist and client collaboratively	The intensity of the emotional experience that it elicits is evaluated	The evaluation is in terms of how it managed to change stance and the narrative	According to developmental stages	Is according to its ability to shift cognitions and to focus on strengths and positive experiences
Research	Collaborate hermeneutic case studies	Case studies and methodologies for intensifying emotional processes and integrating gestalts	Qualitative thematic analyses of content as well as analyses of narrative form according to compositional theories in art and literature	Developmental stages can be studies quantitatively across different populations. Methods for encouraging development can be evaluated	Includes clear measurement of before and after outcomes in regulation, cognition and behaviour
Supervision	Focuses on creating non-judgemental environment and enabling relationship and enhancing creativity through parallel process	Suggestions for methods of working are added, and relationship is also analysed	Ways of working on the story are considered together and analysed	Developmental knowledge is provided and strategies are considered together	Focus on evaluation of progress and methods to enhance progress

Table 9.3 Summary of humanistic theories

	Content	*Composition*	*Therapist*
Humanistic	Conscious	Unconscious	Connector between both levels
Gestalt	Conscious	Unconscious	Connector between both levels
Developmental	Conscious	Unconscious expression of inner developmental level	Encourager of developmental stages of conscious and unconscious levels
Narrative	Conscious	Unconscious	Encourager of shifts in unconscious through content and composition
CBT and mind-body	Conscious standpoints and regulation	Unconscious standpoints and regulation	Shifts from unconscious to conscious

Overall, we see shifts from meaning making in the art, to focusing on positive outcomes in the art. We see influences of existentialism and philosophy, together with influences of behaviourism and science that in the context of postmodern society are mixed together.

In general, the dynamic theories focus on the difference between content and composition. For Freud, content is consciousness, and composition is unconscious; for Jung content is culture, and composition is the universal problems of the psyche; for Winnicott, content and composition are interactive zones where inner and outer reality can meet; and for ego psychology, content is an expression of the power of the ego.

Art therapy shifts from interpreter of art as id, to encourager of artistic processes seeing art as ego, and to initiator of interaction in the art, understanding art as a symbolic zone to enact relationships.

C

ART AS TRANSFORMING SYSTEMS, SOCIETY, THE PRESENT, AND THE FUTURE: ART THROUGH SYSTEMIC THEORIES

We have seen that the theories discussed earlier place the zone of therapeutic inter-action within the individual psyche. The next four theories conceptualize the zone of therapeutic interaction as within the social systems and context in which the individual exists. That is, systemic and social theories assume that the roles and power relations within our families and communities will construct our internal identity. Social theories conceptualize the zone for transformation as situated not only within the individual, but also within the social systems that surround and give form to the individual, such as the ecological circles of family, community, and state, or global systems of power. Within systemic theories, problems are defined as lack of real and social resources due to unjust division of power. Solutions aim to shift roles within systems, to take back both internal and external power and resources, and to actively fight for more power in the system.

The active and confrontational nature of the systemic approach is an important and challenging direction for art therapy, which tends to get caught up with the subjective phenomenology of the individual out of context of the systems that they interact within (Huss, 2012b). In the next chapters, art will be shown to reveal the division of space within the system, framing family or group members from the same social reality as experts. Art will be shown to become a symbolic space within which to define the experience of individual as subject rather than object within a specific social context (Huss and Cwikel, 2008a).

Art is also a space to communicate this with others in the same social reality, and to shift the system through power holders, as a way to visualize new organizations of power. Art will be shown as a tool to gain fresh perspectives and to shake up communication within the system and between cultures. Art enables us to indirectly and non-violently resist or destabilize the existing power relations. Art analysed through a social rather than psychological meta-theory enables power relationships to become visible, and situates art as a culturally contextualized rather than univer-sal language in itself. Thus, whose 'art' dominates art therapy also becomes a power issue. The variations in this theory are outlined in Figure 10.1 and will be explored within the following four chapters.

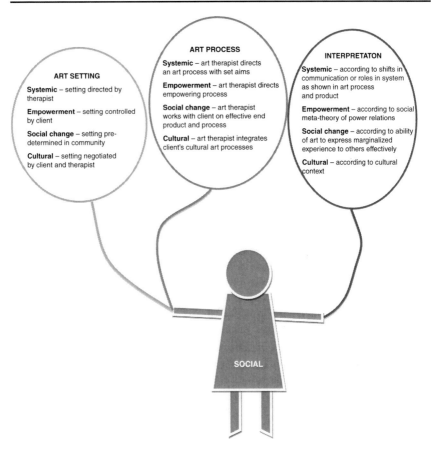

Figure 10.1 Social theories: setting, process, and interpretation

Chapter 10

Art as showing the system
Art therapy and systemic theory

The contribution to art therapy is the overall active, creative, and innovative focus of using art to communicate in the present, explore the past, and shift roles in the here and now through structured symbolic art activities that are based on spatial concepts – a powerful direction for art therapy. The ability of art to simultaneously create a hermeneutic and concrete, and a metaphorical and spatial zone within the system is very helpful. Although art is not often theorized as connected to systemic theories except by a minority of art therapists, art is very relevant to working with systems in that it enables dynamic phenomenological and symbolic expression of the individual within the system.

Systems are complex organisms of interacting parts that cannot be described fully by any single part of the organism. Each change in the system pulls with it a shift in the role of all parts of the system, and redefines the experience of self. For example, if a child remains a problem in school such that it prevents his parents from focusing on their own problems and divorcing, it will not be of help to work with him individually, without understanding the role his behaviour plays within the family system. The homeostatic and power-infused nature of systems seeks stability, but in effect, external factors such as moving country, death, birth, and internal events – for instance, a wish for someone in the system to change – constantly demands an overall shift in the system to incorporate change. Systemic theory is informed by behavioural standpoints that focus on how behaviour changes, rather than on how inner experience changes, assuming that new behaviours in the system will create new experiences. Roles in systems are complementary (victim and aggressor for example) and are not the result of inner conflicts, but rather learnt repetition of roles in the family of origin or as ways to maintain homeostasis in the system. For example, if a woman's mother was battered, she too might marry a battering man, because that is the role she have learnt that enables women to create stability within the system (rather than leaving or challenging) (Mernissi, 2003; Minuchin, 1975; Patterson *et al.*, 2009; Piercy *et al.*, 1996).

The problem is thus defined as having a role within a system that causes suffering or that does not enable individual development or adjustment to changes in the system.

The solution is to change the roles within the system as a whole to meet the needs of individuals in the system or of external changes (such as immigration or death) that the system has to get used to.

The social context of this theory is the rise of sociological theories, behaviourism, and systems theories that affect sciences, social sciences, and humanities (Bandura, 1977; Gladding, 2002; Patterson et al., 2009). Constructivist theories as outlined in the narrative chapter above, dealt with how people within specific contexts construct their reality (Epston, 1996; Payne, 2006).

Micro applications include focusing on the role of the individual within different systems, and of learnt roles even if not working with a whole family or system. The therapy can be based on changing the individual's role in relation to her family, and coping with the resistance of the family to the client's change in role.

The role of art in this theory is that, because systems deal with division of space or resources, art can be seen as a way to concretize the spatial division within the system on account of it being a spatial medium. Often systemic theories shift to visual representations such as diagrams and graphs, as in genograms.

Role of art therapy

Art is also a symbolic medium, and lets us show the organizing metaphors and symbols of the system. Although art is not an inherent part of these theories, the concept of working through symbolic art processes creates new roles in the here and now of the therapy. Art making becomes a methodology for interactive processes. Basically, art is a communicative medium that enables people in conflict to sublimate anger into symbolic forms and thus to communicate their feelings to others without reverting to calcified verbal arguments. Art therefore gives space for all members of the system to express how they experience the system, and to communicate this to others.

Evaluation is based on the observed and reported shifts in roles within the system and the ensuing shifts in the wellbeing of individuals within it. Art will often document the starting roles and also shifts away from them, to new roles and understanding of the system.

Supervision will focus on understanding the system, and on thinking of methods to create change within the system. The focus is solution-oriented and thinking of the role of the therapist in relation to the system, as well as creative ways to reach specific defined aims (Malchiodi and Riley, 1996; Riley and Malchiodi, 1994).

Research will include case studies that analyse family systems and the effectiveness of art interventions. As stated, art becomes a blueprint for the shifts in systems, and on this level can be used as an effective methodology to describe a system and shifts within the system. The aforementioned projective family tests use drawings of family to understand the relationships within the family (Burns, 1987; Riley and Malchiodi, 1994).

Critiquing the theory turns the focus onto shifts in roles, and the impact of the system on the individual that can be seen as disempowering individual agency and individuality from a humanistic perspective. Additionally, in terms of cultural sensitivity, it is a question who decides which roles to shift within the system; in other words, who defines what is a 'healthy' system or family and what is not (Al-Krenawi, 2000; Berry, 1990; Cole, 1996; Gladding, 2002).

Central concepts exemplified through case study

Art as an expression of how an individual experiences the system

Art enables us to define, and then communicate a change in a system in a non-symbolic and thus non-threatening way.

> *When asked to draw each other as symbols, Sharon drew Avital and Shoshana as soft teddy bears that were her 'good mothers' and Rina as a strong soldier. Avital drew all of the women as chicks under her wing expressing her mothering role and older age, but at the end of the group drew them as sisters, protecting her, which showed a shift in her experience of the group space. Sharon was drawn by Rina as a very small child that needed protection at the beginning, relating to her own role as a 'tough' risk taker* (these images are not shown).

Art as an equalizing space in the system

The physical space of the images enables a contained and legitimate space to capture and communicate all experiences of the system.

> *All of the women had visual space to show their images, and verbal space to explain their images. Also Avital explained her lack of image to express her lack of space in her own life through her empty page. This caused the empty page to be an expression of her experience of not existing, rather than acting out a feeling of not existing, not being, through focusing on others than on self.*

Exploring the family of origin through images

The values, roles, culture, and history of the family of origin are internalized by each person in order to challenge them. These values first have to be made manifest, and art helps to concretize the reality (e.g. 'my father drank') and the experience of the reality (e.g. 'I always had to protect my mother').

> *Avital created an image of lines of clean washing. She stated that in her family the most important thing was not to let outsiders know that there were problems. Dirty washing was always kept inside and everyone was silent about what was happening with her alcoholic father inside the house. She decided to talk to her daughters about her past sexual abuse to break the 'clean washing' mode of interaction* (not shown).

Art as a symbolic process within which to capture and change roles

The art process is a symbolic and controlled zone within which people interact and their style of interaction can be 'caught' on the page. Once the role (such as leader, rescuer, or criticizer) is identified, the art process can be modified to create a new role.

> *Each woman was given a colour and asked to draw together on the same page without talking. In the first image Avital added and strengthened everyone else's parts in the image but did not have any space for drawing herself. In the second round of combined drawing, the art therapist instructed Avital to take a space and create her own image there, trusting the rest of the group to manage without her help* (not shown).

Working the theory: art therapy skills and techniques

Verbal techniques

The systemic or family therapist has a 'tool box' of interventions similar to a plumber whose job it is to help shake up and reorganize the plumbing of a system. Strategies include: first, to understand the roles within the system; second, to connect these roles to the family of origin; third, to enable better communication within the family; and last, most importantly, to encourage shifts in roles in the here and now of the therapy and at home.

These stages demand an active role for the therapist to change a system which prefers to stay static. 'Homework' is set to practise new roles and new ways of interacting. Active manipulations of the existing order, using confrontations, behavioural suggestions, metaphors, and paradoxical interventions can be used. At this level, the therapist activates new behaviours and new perspectives, and confronts old perspectives.

Visual techniques

Setting

Art is usually utilized in directive ways, to create different symbolic experiences within a manipulated setting. For example, clients can use fluid materials for merging a disengaged system, or use dry materials for creating boundaries in a symbiotic system. The art work can focus on emotions, organization, or communication, according to what the therapist thinks will help change the system. The therapy space needs to be large enough to enable combined art work, and the materials diverse enough to create different types of experiences; but the art therapist monitors the materials and aims to direct and orchestrate the art use.

Process

Art therapists can, as shown above, use art as communication. For example, everyone can draw how they experience the move to a new city. The page equalizes the spaces of adults, children, and dominant and non-dominant parts of the family in that each has a personal space of the same size on the page.

Art may also be used to concretize spatial relationships, and to express the roles within the system. For example, the family may draw a picture together and see how decisions and space were negotiated. Additionally the art therapist may shift the interaction within the system, through directing roles, for example, by creating a game where the family creates an image in which the mother is passive and the father interacts with the children. The art therapist thus harnesses her creativity to initiate and direct art interventions within the present time of the group. She is able to creatively improvise an activity that becomes a method to reach a shift in perception or behaviour or interaction within the system. The art is directive, aiming to create a new experience, in a metaphorical and thus less threatening way. For example, a single mother with authority problems may be instructed to direct an art activity for her children (Huss, 2008; Kerr and Hoshino, 2008; Riley and Malchiodi, 1994).

Another use is to explore the family of origin through images as a way to concretize their presence and impact. Settings and art materials are subsumed to the specific aims of the types of systematic changes that the therapist aims to make.

Art interpretation

Art interpretation is based on the spatial relationships, relative sizes, and overall interactions between the different elements portrayed in the art. For example, who is left out of a family drawing, who is most central, who is smallest or furthest away, or who is next to the client. This becomes a formalized method of analysing a family, as seen in Burns' family series of drawings (Burns, 1987). A less formal method might include observing family interaction around an art activity, and observing the effectiveness of the art as a method to enable shifts in communication and roles, as well as perceptions of roles from the family of origin.

Overall skills to practise

- *Identify roles* such as scapegoat, leader, coalitions in the system, distracter, and identify who has the power to initiate change in the system through joint art pictures and history of the family.
- *Identify how each person in the system experiences the system.*
- *Communicate this to each other*, making space and legitimacy for all.
- *Identify a central set of values of the system*, and create a metaphor to make it visible.
- *Use your creativity to create games that shift the above identified roles* and communication patterns, and help to create new leaders and coalitions in the system.
- *Work on the family of origin of adults* in the system using creative genograms.

Art-based skills to practise

- Draw a creative genogram of your family, showing central themes and roles of the family through symbols, colours, and shapes over the generations as you experience them.
- Draw your family as different fish in the sea, or as animals in the zoo, or create a sculpture of your family. Draw the objects but also the surroundings (what kind of sea is it; what type of zoo).
- Draw a group picture in which each person uses one colour and you are not allowed to talk. Afterwards each person analyses their own role within the picture, in relation to other roles on the page. Discuss the role you took on the page in connection to the image of the family of origin.
- Draw another picture together using the same colour in which you consciously shift to a new role, and then discuss how it felt to adopt a new role.
- Draw a symbol of someone in your family that concerns you. Draw a symbol of yourself, and a bridge between you both. Enact a dialogue between you.
- If needed, create a dialogue, separation ritual, or other representation of mourning, or shift in the relationship from your side.
- Draw a present for everyone in your family and imagine what each person would give you.

Chapter 11

Art as claiming space

Art therapy and empowerment

This theory's contribution to art therapy is that art as a basic communicative language enables marginalized groups to first identify what is lacking, and second, to communicate this to others. It can intensify the interpretive and negotiating voice of the client and thus return both internal and external power. This is a powerful use of art that is always a meeting between the individual and the social context, or between figure and background. On the one hand, one can say that people don't need art when they have such unmet basic needs. On the other, art may help to self-define areas of power, resources and spiritual and emotional strengths in order to prepare to undertake the battle for survival from a disempowered stance. Art can be used to map out issues, think of solutions, and organize resources, as well as to express feelings (Freire and Macedo, 1987; Saulnier, 1996). Most importantly, the therapist can use art to connect between social theories and subjective experience.

Although there is much discussion of social art therapy contexts in art therapy literature (e.g. community art, social change, and art in disaster work or in institutions), the application of social critical theories still remains marginal within art therapy theory, which is informed by universal psychological and humanistic theories rather than by social critical theories. However, art contexts such as the many art therapy clients in the public sphere (e.g. schools, community centres, and health and psychiatric institutions) have a high representation of marginalized and non-hegemonic social groups. Art therapy clients in the public sector are often affected by immigration, poverty, and other social problems. Therefore a social perspective is particularly relevant and imperative within art therapy training.

Empowerment theories, in continuation of the systemic theories already discussed, focus on different roles within the systems, and on the power relationships of these roles within larger social systems. The theory of empowerment assumes that all relationships are power imbued, and assumes that the ecological layers that comprise the socio-cultural context of the client's reality can include different types of disempowerment and marginalization, such as racial, gendered, or ethnic lack of power. This creates personal pain: thus, the political becomes the personal.

Critical social theories understand power as a dynamic and relative construct that is at the base of all social interactions, and that shapes personal experience. In accordance with Foucault's concept of power, power relationships are built into all systems, and all types of relationship, in a dynamic, relative, and evolving way. In light of this, the relationship between client and therapist is by definition power-infused on different levels such as race, culture, gender, etc. These power relations construct the therapeutic relationship and need to be dismantled to create an experience of empowerment within the here and now of the therapeutic relationship (Foucault, 2000). The social context that constructs self is power infused along different interactive parameters – thus, a woman can be marginalized at the level of gender, culture, and ethnicity, and these different types of marginalization will all interact within a specific socio-cultural reality at a given time. Marginalization stems from social and economic policies that create systematic discrimination and deprivation based on race, ethnicity, religion, or gender, exacerbated by processes of immigration, war, and political instability as well as general social disorganization and conflicting values within the social system.

The problem is lack of power both in terms of resources and in terms of internalized helplessness, disempowerment, and impoverishment of self. This is due to unequal distribution of power in society, and active oppression or discrimination.

The solution is not only to shift roles but also to actively fight to take back power through raising awareness of the forms of social oppression one is experiencing, as well as strategies to reclaim one's power internally and within personal and social interactions. This demands first creating insight into the implications of this disempowerment; second, locating the problem within society rather than within the individual's own psyche; and third, exploring areas where power might be reclaimed. This process de-pathologizes the client, enabling him to understand himself as a victim of a lack of social power, rather than as inherently flawed or weak, as found in paternalistic or fatalistic narratives about poverty (Alcock, 1997; Brington and Lykes, 1996). Another aim of this type of therapy is to refer the client to people who can give information regarding services, rights, and physical help, and who are considered part of the therapeutic relationship, if these are what the client defines as his problems (Saulnier, 1996). Thus another facet of power is information (Freire and Macedo, 1987; Saulnier, 1996; Wandersman and Florin, 2003; Zimmerman, 2000).

The social context of these theories includes postmodern and critical social thinking, such as Foucault's conception that power permeates all relationships but is unequally distributed. This ideological stance has a clear social agenda that aims to resist global and neo-capitalist social organization, which keeps power among a privileged few, and that discounts specific social context and reality as a way of oppressing people. While psychology aims to adjust people to oppressive realities, this social theory aims to adjust the reality so that people are not oppressed and do not develop the symptoms of oppression, discrimination, and marginalization (Alcock, 1997; Bronner, 2011; Foucault, 2000; Jameson, 1991).

Micro applications are that empowerment is often undertaken in groups as a way to create narratives of the reality experienced by a group of people with similar types of social oppressions; then empowerment interventions, as stated, assume that individual experience is always political, and thus the individual's problems can be analysed according to the above meta-theories of power – as in feminist therapy. The power relationships between client and therapist are also explored as part of this.

The role of art is, as stated in Chapter 10 at a systemic level, that art enables one to see divisions of space and power relations. Space ownership is always a power issue. Therefore showing a lack of space becomes a way to resist lack of space. Art also expresses the experience of the individual as the subject, not the object. This is important for marginalized groups who do not usually have the power to self-define themselves and their experience is defined from the outside. The visual concept of the 'gaze' points to the power of who gazes at or defines whom. Creative expression is thus empowering as it becomes a way to self-define identity as well as a way to gaze back at society and to name what is seen.

Additionally, verbal expression is often the terminology of the dominant groups, and so a shift to non-verbal expression enables one to redefine the concepts of the discourse. For example, Spivak and Guha (1988) claim that the history of women in the developing world can be found in aesthetic texts, rather than in historical literature. They argue that history and intellectualism have remained male areas and that there is a lack of room for women's voices. Thus, literature and art, which are not bonded to dominant ideologies concerning reality – such as history, politics, and other power structures – allow the expression of marginalized voices (Foster, 2007; Freire and Macedo, 1987; Hooks, 1992; Huss and Cwikel, 2007, 2008a; Jameson, 1991; Jones, 2003; Joughin and Maples, 2004; Lippard, 1990; Soja, 1989; Spivak and Guha, 1988).

However, according to the humanistic stance, art is often assumed to bridge these power relations by shifting to a visual mode that is considered 'universal' or that skips the power bases of language (Campbell, 1999a; Hiscox and Calisch, 1998) But, from a critical stance, art itself, like everything else, is embedded within and is an expression of power relationships. For example, crafts, which are in effect female art forms, are often considered 'lower' than fine art (Jones, 2003; Lippard, 1995). Art therapists are therefore in danger of imposing their understandings of art on the client (Hogan, 2003; Huss, 2008, 2009b, 2012a, 2013). Knowledge, or the ability to define art issues, is always power infused. Thus, art therapists have power over defining the problem of their client when, for example, using a diagnostic art test, or when interpreting art work as in the humanistic theories (see Chapter 1). This turns the client into the object and the therapist into the expert about both art and the client (Wadeson, 2000). Reclaiming knowledge by defining and interpreting one's experience as the subject is a way of taking back power. Art, as a phenomenological tool, enables us to intensify the self-expression, but also self-definition of our knowledge about different issues, and their interpretation, as long as the creator of the art is the central interpreter. This connects to basic premises within the humanistic standpoints as well (Hogan, 1997, 2003; Huss, 2009a; 2011, 2012a).

According to feminism in the developing world, identity can be broken down into interacting levels of oppression, which might include culture, ethnicity, gender, and poverty. These interact in different ways within different social realities. For example, a young woman may wish to remain a traditional wife, but suffer from poverty. Art may help to break down these different elements of identity by creating a multifaceted and flexible space in which to express different parts of oneself – as in gestalt theories. This can break down static and reductionist definitions of self, and also point to spaces of agency in the gaps between different types of oppressions (Mohanty, 2003).

The role of the art therapist is to utilize art as a method to, first of all, give back the power of defining the content of the empty page, because the creator has absolute power over what and how to depict on the page, and then, how to interpret it. This symbolic reclaiming of power may be used to 'dare to imagine' a new way of interacting, and to plan for real life changes that bring back power to the client. The therapists also use social meta-theories of power to analyse the verbalizations and art of the client, to show how power relationships impact on the client's personal suffering.

Evaluation in this type of therapy is ongoing and collaborative. The art therapist can more or less evaluate the use of power in relation to and in interaction with herself, as well as in the client's life, from a position that is more powerful.

Art evaluation is not structured but can reveal empowerment by taking up more space, self-defining issues through art, making choices in the art process, and by situating problems within a social reality in terms of the background – subject relationship – and in terms of the art's content. There will be other emerging manifestations of power within the art content, composition, process, and product.

Supervision focuses on analysing all elements of the therapy according to a social meta-narrative, in terms of division of power; in terms of empowerment practices, verbally and in art; and in terms of imparting knowledge. The paradox of being the 'expert' and imparting knowledge through a social-critical-analytical prism, but empowering the client to think for herself and to be her own expert, is addressed within the supervision in terms of parallel processes, and may be explored through art making.

Research aims to destabilize power relationships between researcher and researchee by shifting to visual expression. As in empowerment therapy, the aim of using art within this type of research is to intensify the interpretive voice of the participant as part of a non-dominant group. The research participant, like the client, becomes in effect the expert on his or her own experience. This enables them to destabilize hegemonic verbal conceptions of issues, such as terminologies used by researchers, and to shift to the knowledge definitions of the participants themselves. On this level, then, therapy itself becomes a type of participatory action research method, in which client and therapist collaboratively research the impact of social reality on subjective experience, and the impact of the therapy on the client, with the aim of sharing knowledge. Thus, the distance between empowerment and art-based research aims and methods is small and often overlapping (Foster, 2007; Gerken, 2001; Huss *et al.*, 2011; Knowles and Cole, 2008: Lawler, 2002; Tuhiwai-Smith, 1999).

A critique of this theory is that if used to portray the client as a victim of social oppression, it might encourage helplessness, in that the client blames the system rather than focuses on solutions. Another problem could be, as with dynamic theories, that focusing on a rigid meta-theory limits additional understanding of an issue, such as deep defences, or the importance of subjective experience. It may also limit the possibility of a person to self-actualize even under conditions of disempowerment. Another problem is the paradox of imposing a social critical meta-theory on a disempowered client, as stated above.

Central concepts exemplified through case study

Integrating personal versus social interpretations as empowerment

Issues of interpretation are always power infused, as knowledge is power. Thus, in empowerment theories, the client alone initially interprets the art work, and then, interpretation might be according to a theory of social power, provided by the therapist. An example of these two interpretations follows.

> Rina stated that her (abusive) boyfriend was good for her, and that she wanted to stay with him, while the therapist analysed his behaviour as disempowering for her. She suggested that Rina define if he was in the 'black or colourful' side of her image (B2, B1). Rina stated that he was in the black which made him exciting. The therapist suggested she drew the boyfriend's advantages and disadvantages, and also related his personality to male roles in her creative genogram of family of origin.
>
> The group also worked with magazines that showed images of women as helpless. The mandala that Rina drew (B4) enabled her to conceive of herself as both strong and weak, rather than needing a 'strong' but abusive boyfriend to feel protected or to experience her femininity. The connection between femininity and weakness was broken. All of this helped Rina to understand the implication of giving up her power by staying with her boyfriend. Eventually she decided to leave him when she had connected to other inner strengths.

Creating art as an internal reclamation of power; and using art to influence and communicate with others

> The group poster initiated by Avital (D3) was empowering on many levels. First, on the level of the composition and content, it showed the power of the group that is contained within a flowerpot. It reframed the women as flowers, symbolizing purity and growth as opposed to the 'damaged goods' stigmas that sexually abused women often have to deal with from society, and that become internalized. Avital's use of the poster to lecture

frames the women survivors as experts who can inform others, which is empowering. In addition, breaking the silence and visually speaking out, is in itself an empowering act, since it gives voice and visibility to an experience that might create shame.

Using a group to challenge social standpoints

Shoshana (A) was a religious woman, and explained that there was much pressure on her to have a baby within her culture as part of her gendered role and the central achievement of women. Thus the social pressure was cultural, religious, and gendered. When looking at her images, she could define these different pressures to have a baby before she was ready. She decided to wait until she felt ready.

Rina wanted to find out about her rights so that she could leave her unsatisfying 'tough' job as a guard. The art therapist put her in contact with a community service agent who could help her find a new job and define her rights from the old job.

Analysing art through social rather psychological theories as part of consciousness raising

In one session the women used images of women from magazines to explore their female identity, while also drawing images of themselves. They analysed the impact of the magazine images that objectified women – as images that were internalized by them, but that they didn't agree with.

Using the page to explore internal sources of power

We saw that Avital first addressed her lack of self and lack of power on the page, and second, reclaimed her anger through art, and used this as the power to develop a poster to be used in social activism.

Working the theory: art therapy skills and techniques

Verbal skills

According to this theory, therapists need to hold an ideological world view that does not accept paternalistic understandings of poverty being on account of clients' inherent weaknesses, which would disempower their clients, rather than it being because of the social structural division of power. As already stated, the role of the therapist is to *raise the client's awareness of different types of social marginalization that have impacted her or his problems*, based on social meta-theories. In addition to this internal process of consciousness raising, the therapist helps the client to identify ways in which the client devolves power, or has internalized lack of power, in interaction with both the therapist and with others. This may include efforts to change self-defeating behaviours, and to change power relations within intimate relationships, within the community, and within society as a whole, through social change and activism.

A zone for enacting this is in the relationship with the therapist. The therapist actively explores power relations and cultural and social standpoints as manifest in the relationship between the client and the therapist (where, by definition, the therapist has more power as the 'expert' and is often from the hegemonic social group). The danger of this that the client might remain within the victim identity and hopelessness, where society is blamed for his problems and agency reduced. The therapist is thus the opposite of a 'blank screen' and gives up power in relation to the client by explaining cultural assumptions, training, and other self-characteristics, as well as assuming that the client can define if the therapy is helping. The therapist also imparts useful information that can help the client regain power, such as her social rights, relevant resources in the community, reading material and others.

A group format as often chosen as it enables a group of people suffering from the same types of social oppression or marginalization to see that the problem is shared, and thus not individual, and enables sharing of knowledge and resources to fight back. The therapist's stance is to treat group members as experts in their social problems, rather than herself and to encourages the group to self-define problems and solutions (Freire and Macedo, 1987; Huss, 2007, 2008, 2010, 2011; Liebmann, 1994; Saulnier, 1996).

Visual techniques

Setting

The setting can be varied. There could be a focus on words, with art used as a way to illustrate and trigger verbalizations, or to intensify ideas and subjective experience (Hogan, 1997, 2003; Liebmann, 2003). Conversely, art as an inherently empowering experience of taking up time and space for exploring the self, demands a more open studio setting with a range of materials and safety to enable this process.

Art process

Overall, the verbalizations around art include the inherently empowering element of self-definition in creating an image, as well as the interpretive element of explaining an image. The therapist often uses a social meta-theory of power or gender to analyse the image. The aim is to utilize art for the exploration of identity in relation to social reality. The art is self-directed by the client so as not to impose the therapist's power. For example, if a client wants to make something decorative, or is concerned with the product, then the therapist considers how not to impose her aesthetic values of what is art on to the client.

Interpretation of the art

Interpretation operates according to its empowering role for the client (e.g. by the client being able to self-define her experience and needs on the empty page). The analytical prism is according to the social meta-theory of unequal distribution of power, as expressed in content, composition, process, and interpretation of the art work. The art therapist may thus actively interpret the image in a different way from that of the client (e.g. pointing to how white women are portrayed in the image as more attractive than black women). Analysing art through social theories rather than through psychological theories becomes a methodology of consciousness raising. As stated, a central role of therapy from an empowerment perspective is to raise consciousness of power relationships and of ways that one has been disempowered. Art is therefore often analysed as personal and subjective, rather than as located within and expressing a specific social reality.

Overall skills to practise

- *Taking client's social or real-world challenges seriously as part of the therapy* and not focusing only on subjective emotional reality.
- *Using art to create a connection between the social and the subjective levels of experience* and of reality.
- *Actively teaching clients to analyse their art through social theories* with prisms of class, gender, and culture.
- *At the same time positioning clients as the experts of their own experience* by enabling their expressive and interpretive power to be the first analytical strategy.
- *Overtly addressing issues of power* in understanding of art within the therapy sessions.
- *Identifying strategies and planning for ways to reclaim power through art*, first in the symbolic zone of the art, and second in relation to real life by becoming knowledgeable about services and self-help groups in the area, and actively collaborating with them.

Art-based skills to practise

- Create an image of a current problem that you are dealing with and analyse it according to gender, class, and culture. Try to understand the problem in the context of these issues.
- Analyse existing images in advertising, or in your visual culture, for their social messages, as expressed within the compositional elements. Use these as a starting point for art, which becomes a personal statement.
- Learn about social services empowerment and self-help groups in the area in which you practise art therapy; make contact with someone who can inform you and your clients.
- Learn about social and activist artists; explore an issue that is of importance to you personally and become socially active in relation to it, aiming to use art to express your activism.

Chapter 12

Art as a space to fight
Art therapy and social theories

Social change, in continuation of the earlier empowerment chapter, claims that if the problem lies in an oppressive society rather than in the individual, the solution is to change society rather than the individual. Dynamic and humanistic orientations can be critiqued as aiming to cajole the clients into adjusting to the status quo, rather than creating a social reality where the individual has real power and possibility to solve their problems. This viewpoint situates the therapist not as a perpetuator of a social system, but as at the forefront of engaging clients to fight the system. Taking back power in reality can be defined as the most 'therapeutic' act in that one can impact oness surroundings.

The aim is to change the status quo, influence power holders and public opinion, and create more real resources for those who need them. This is often expressed in self-help and advocacy groups as well as in social change forums. This is different from a paternalistic stance of raising money to help communities or individuals as in philanthropy, as it does not aim to redistribute social resourses or to actively change society. Neither does it engage the people who need help in the struggle to receive resources that will help solve problems and change opinions (Alcock, 1997; Bronner, 2011; Jameson, 1991; Kvale, 1992; Martin and Sugarman, 2000; Miller, 1996; Spivak and Guha, 1988; Zimmerman, 2000).

The problem can be defined as an unjust oppressive social order that creates a lack of basic resources for some. The solution is to fight to change various standpoints in society in order to redistribute resources in a fairer way, by mobilizing clients to take social action and become a resource for themselves, and to advocate change in the standpoints of power holders.

The social context of this theory, as covered in the empowerment chapter, is the influence of social-critical theories on psychology and on the art world. Interestingly there is a movement within fine art that wishes to move away from the elitism of galleries, and of critics, wishing to reconnect with communities and to impact on social reality. This is a place of conversion for social art therapists and social artists. However, these directions are still basically different because their theoretical orientations – and therefore aims – are different. Artists want to create interesting art, while social art therapists want to engage communities in art as empowerment and to impact standpoints (Harrington, 2004; Hills, 2001; Lippard 1995).

Micro applications apply this theory to individual therapy, in that the 'personal is political' as well: while social change demands interaction and collaboration with groups to advocate social change, activism is an individual choice that can become part of individual empowerment and can strongly impact on society, as exemplified by individual activists who catch media attention and change viewpoints.

The role of art, as stated in Chapters 10 and 11 on systemic and empowerment theories, is making oppression visible to those who experience it and to those who enable it, and hence becomes the first step in fighting it. Hegemonic discourse often hides social injustice under abstract concepts that camouflage how power has been taken away. Art shifts the discourse to a visual one, and reveals how the power has been taken away. The use of art as communication, as a way to arouse the senses, challenge cognitions, and create engagement in a non-violent and indirect way makes it an excellent medium to manifest other's suffering (Huss and Maor, 2015; Landgarten, 2013; Moon, 2003; Naumberg, 1966; Rogers, 2007). If direct documentation is too traumatic to internalize, then art enables a more indirect and less flooding type of engagement with the suffering of others. For example, Butler (2001) describes artists' projects involving social issues through the metaphor of 'waves', where the ripples touch and vibrate around an issue and the art becomes a 'silent witness' to injustice. Because art is not real but symbolic, it can mimic systems, and thus reveal power systems. In other words, because art itself participates in semblances of illusions, it highlights these qualities of taken-for-granted illusions that disempower (Alcock, 1997; Harrington, 2004; Hills, 2001; Jameson, 1991; Jones, 2003; Shank, 2005; Spivak, 1988). The transformative powers of images to change stance are well understood within advertising and other fields using images to indirectly influence people on a macro level. Likewise, art can also be used to shift social consensus, as in social activist art movements (Huss, 2013; Kalmanowitz and Lloyd, 2005; Kaplan, 2006; Levine and Levine, 2011; Orr, 2007; Speiser and Speiser, 2007).

The art therapist's role is that their active knowledge of art methods and art and community connections enable clients to use art within the public sphere to advocate changes of opinion – and raise awareness of issues. This requires having community, political, and art knowledge, as well as connections. The aim is not to create 'high art' but community projects that involve the community while also impacting the surroundings (Huss, 2012a, 2012b, 2013; Kalmanowitz and Lloyd, 2005; Kaplan, 2006; Levine and Levine, 2011; Orr, 2007; Speiser and Speiser, 2007).

Supervision should include active focusing on the aims, strategies, and expected as well as unexpected outcomes of the project. The supervisor is a more experienced social activist and shares his or her knowledge and contacts, acting as a guide and mentor for the overall process.

Research in this type of art intervention starts with researching the context and wished-for outcome, therefore by definition it is a type of participatory research project. Often the art product itself is the outcome of this research, as in documentaries. The concept of participatory research is central to art in social change. In addition to the aim of monitoring and evaluating these projects together with the community, social research concepts claim that research must not only benefit the community's knowledge, or the researcher's, but must also have a transformative and social change element in itself, in order to improve the problems of the participants. Art-based research claims that art enables this through creating a communicative end product, which tells the story and impacts those observing it, shifting the discourse of the research away from abstract verbal thinking to a method that directly defines and interacts with the issue (Foster, 2007; Gerken, 2001; Huss, 2011, 2012b; Knowles and Cole, 2008; Lawler, 2002; Tuhiwai-Smith, 1999).

A critique of this theory could be that it encourages a focus on external elements rather than internal processes of change, and is therefore not really therapy. As for empowerment theories, it uses a rigid social meta-theory that may limit additional understandings of the issue. When artists are involved, another problem is that the line between art as aesthetic product and art as social change is often blurred. It is not always clear if the artist, or art therapist, or the community benefit in terms of credit from the final art product. As stated in Chapter 11, while there are many books on art and social change, they are often based in altruistic paternalistic and humanistic theories that do not really empower the clients or provide a social critical frame for understanding the intervention or the art. The focus is often on the general contribution of self-expression to health resilience and trauma management for marginalized populations in crises. This does not engage with utilizing art to seriously challenge and transform society.

Contributions to art therapy are in effect based on the above described challenges of this stance. Often art therapists struggle to stay within the 'clinical' definition of their work; however, the ability to define art use in a broader socially oriented direction enables art therapists to become genuinely active in the community and in social change, using their very relevant art and therapy skills. Art enables clients to connect phenomenological experience to social reality, and this enables the scope of art therapy to be extended. It does not have to be dramatic, but can include art therapists, in collaboration with art teachers, to fight against stigma and for social change campaign projects and exhibitions in schools for example, rather than insisting that they are 'clinical' and stay behind closed doors. It forces them to engage with the effect of the art product on society, and the ensuing political and social issues that it raises. This returns the energy of art as communication and as a way to transform the world, not just individuals, through art therapy. With the advent of privatized healthcare, many groups of people suffering from problems have no choice but to rely on themselves and to become active and advocate their needs. Art therapists have much to contribute to these groups.

Central concepts as demonstrated in the case study

Participatory action

> The group poster (D4) became a strategy to raise awareness of an issue that is silenced in society, and to advocate more serious punishment for sexual offenders. It raised

empathy because of its positive motif of flowers, and was therefore not too painful to observe.

Planning the project's different stages

The art therapist connected the women to a graphic designer and printers who were prepared to donate their skills and resources to help create the poster. They planned the image together, thinking of all of its meanings, but also how to make an effective statement while maintaining the women's privacy by using only parts of images.

Planning for visibility

The women in the group who initiated the poster rang up many community centres, prisons, and the municipality court house to suggest displaying a poster and making a lecture about it. The poster did not stand alone as a fine art work, but was used as a visual trigger for further communication around the issue.

Utilizing multi-model interventions to capture media attention

In continuation of the above, the women connected to a local dance group and did a gig that included a 'dance for women's right to move freely' initiative. The use of multi-model art directions intensified the impact of the message and created more collaboration.

The local rape crisis centre created a special fund-raising event and used the poster to advertise it. They invited singers who donated their time and crafts, and suggested that it be a 'dance for women's right to move freely'.

Working the theory: art therapy skills and techniques

Verbal techniques

According to this viewpoint, therapists who utilize a fatalistic understanding of poverty as the result of the client's inherent weaknesses, or as an inevitable way of organizing society that puts the most vulnerable at the bottom, are by definition disempowering clients, because they conceptualize the client's problems as due to their inherent weakness rather than social oppression (Alcock, 1997; Brington and Lykes, 1996).

A social understanding of problems, as opposed to a pathological understanding, in itself can be therapeutic because the blame is attributed to a social context rather than to the individual (e.g. a women who suffers from domestic violence might understand that it is not that she is weak, but that society enables men to be violent to women with little punishment). In addition to this internal process of consciousness raising that was described in the earlier chapter, in the social change context, the therapist helps the client to identify active strategies to gain power and to change standpoints within day-to-day life. The therapist is thus the opposite of a 'blank screen', is an active collaborator and someone with knowledge of and connections within the community and politics. The art therapist has to create political and social networks and visibility. The art therapist therefore has to become 'political' in effect, in order to impact the political zone and to utilize art for the above described exploration of identity in relation to social reality.

As stated, the role of the therapist is to raise the client's awareness of different types of social marginalization that have affected her problems. A group format is often chosen as it enables a group of people, suffering from the same types of social oppression or marginalization, to see that the problem is shared, is not individual, which enables a sharing of knowledge and treating group members as experts in their social problems – rather than the therapist. This can then be communicated to power holders and used to advocate rights, for example, in self-help groups.

Visual techniques

Setting

Settings may focus on simple art materials, such as felt-tip pens, to self-define and express one's experiences to others. Conversely, structured art projects will take the art out of the therapy or studio into the community; therefore art materials and art expertise will be utilized as in an art studio. Art products are often made within and connected to the community, such as the community centre, or a park where the art making and product will be visible to all, or taken out of the setting and made and exhibited elsewhere. The community as a whole becomes the setting of the art intervention, creating many networks and connections within the community as a positive side effect.

Art process

This involves actively researching the needs of the community and identifying areas of intervention as self-defined by the community themselves. This type of collaborative research ensures that the art activity will address real needs rather than those imposed by the therapist (Zimmerman, 2000).

The next stage will be to translate this into a visual project with the dual aim of an empowering process and a communicative product. For example, the art therapist may provide cameras for a group of girls to photograph the best and worst places in their slum neighbourhood. This helps to reframe the area as holding positive elements for the girls, – which are internalized into their self-identity. Eventually, the exhibition may be sent to the town authorities and to the local papers to encourage clean-up and safety in the area, it being the most negative point that the girls photographed in their area (Huss, 2012a). Another example is in the exemplifying case study of this book, in which images of sexually abused women are used to create a poster to raise awareness and to demand more intense punishment for abusers. Another example is a group of teenagers in a drug-infested area creating a sculpture park of the advantages (on one side of the sculpture park) and the disadvantages (on the other side) of taking drugs. This enables the teenagers to explore the issue for themselves, and also for other youths who come to the park to see it. It also creates a park for the community's use (Huss, 2012a). Another example is putting up pictures of 'local heroes' in a community to empower the community to take further action.

Art interpretation

This is a form of evaluation that reaches the two goals of empowerment and social impact. The art does not become an art product that stands alone as in fine art, but is rather a trigger for agency, activity, dialogue, and media attention. On this level it remains an art therapy product that gains meaning through dialogue with the producer of the art, even if it is exhibited and stands 'alone' from the therapist or client.

Art interpretation is defined according to the success of the project in creating social change and mobilizing awareness, changing standpoints, and intensifying power and coping methods of those suffering from the problem – art is a means to an end, rather than an end in itself. Overall, the impact of social change is hard to measure in the short term, as its reverberations are in many directions and long term. However, in accordance with social theories, it is important to make every effort to try to evaluate the outcome and impact of the project as a whole, from the perspective of different stakeholders who define the various elements of the project. Art therapists can focus on the group processes, empowerment factors, and impact of the final project as manifest in process and in product.

Overall skills to practise

- *Researching self-defined community needs* through art-based participatory methods.
- *Becoming 'political'* Understanding stakeholders, power holders, and the interests of those involved.
- *Creating a committed group of activists.*
- *Creating community coalitions and coalitions* with power holders and with community artists.
- *Planning an intervention strategy together with the community* and planning the use of art according to this.
- *Exploring the empowerment and social impact characteristics of the art project.*
- *Utilizing senses and aesthetics to enhance visibility,* and creating a multi-model methodology to enhance visibility.
- *Creating relevant media coverage and documentation of the art event* and systematically assessing its impact on the community.

Art-based skills to practise

- Think of a situation where you feel lack of power.
- Express this lack of power in art.
- Analyse how you could change the situation and get more power, and who you would have to influence; create an art work for that person.
- Find community and social change activists and artists in your local area and study their processes and end products.
- Analyse an advertising campaign that is popular right now and define their messages and strategies, as well as how to subvert it to a social message.
- Join a group that cares about something that you also care about.

Chapter 13

Art as cultural values

Art therapy and culture

This theory's contribution to art therapy is that art therapy includes a search for places where people create images that are meaningful for them, which implies connecting between art therapy and cultural contexts, rather than encapsulating the client within a psychological space disconnected from her use of images. This suggests a rich theoretical prism for art therapy, because culture is expressed in art. It enables art therapy to become more involved in the world and in art on a real contextualized level and challenges central art therapy ideologies of expressivity, individualism, universal psychic constructs as expressed in composition, and focuses on the process rather than on the product (McNiff, 1998).

It also challenges the assumption that art has to occur within the closed space of the therapy room in order to be therapy, rather than, for example, within a temple, in a community setting, or in front of the television. Putting culture at a deep level within art therapy helps to diversify art therapy from a global reductionist understanding of culture, to culture as an intense source of power within art therapy.

Cultural theories define all systems – families, groups, and communities, as well as therapy – as creating and existing within different sets of cultural values that inform and organize the systems. Therapy is defined in this book as a socio-cultural construct that reacts to a specific social context, defining what is a problem and what is a solution through this culturally contextualized lens. Indeed, in many cultures the concept of therapy does not exist as a separate entity, but occurs in different contexts such as religious, familial, or educational interaction. Clearly, because therapy and art therapy are Western concepts, using Western understandings of what is therapy and what is art, all of the ideas outlined in the earlier chapters may not be relevant to other cultures. To complicate the issue even further, culture itself is not a static concept, but one that includes religion, ethnicity, location, class, social power, and different combinations of the above. Thus, people from the same ethnicity but different social levels of power may be more different in terms of culture than those from the same social class but from different ethnicities; or a man may have a different cultural conditioning to a woman in the same culture and feel more comfortable with a man from a different culture (Hocoy, 2002).

In light of this, the concept of universality that is central to Western psychological theories is in itself problematic. If the cultural norm is individuation and development of inner locus of control, as in Western culture, then a mother and daughter who are dependent on each other will be considered pathological, whereas in a collective culture, mother and daughter may be expected to work as part of an intimate team, that is perhaps more intimate than husband and wife. Shifting roles of communicating and of coping are also culturally defined; for example, in many cultures, a parent who does not hit their child to discipline it does not love their child, while in Western society, it is not acceptable to hit a child. Thus, differences in culture are also power imbued in terms of what is defined as normative and what is not. The meeting between two cultures is usually a meeting between a dominant culture (the therapist) and a marginal culture (the client).

To further complicate the issue, most people in today's globalized society belong to at least two different cultures simultaneously, and have a hybrid definition of culture. Thus, a definition of a client's culture from the 'outside' holds the danger of being a reductionist stance which does not fit the client's reality. For example, dichotomies between Western versus non-Western, collective versus individualized, and traditional versus modern cultures as used above, simplify what is, in effect, a spectrum (Al-Krenawi, 2000; Berry, 1990; Cole, 1996; Dwairy, 2004; Hobfoll, 2001; Kaplan, 2000; Mohanty, 2003; Said, 1978; Spivak and Guha, 1988; Sue, 1996).

One problem with this theory is the lack of cultural understanding between therapist and client of what constitutes a problem and a solution. An answer is to try to negotiate these different cultural understandings and to reach a solution that expresses the understandings of the dominant culture and of the clients' culture.

In light of the relativist and social theories that stress the influence of social power systems and their values on the individual, rather than assuming a universal theory that in effect imposes a Western world view on all as in global society, culture is understood as an important construct within therapy (Foucault, 2000; Gerken, 2001).

In all of the above cultural power complexities are present within art use in therapy because, as Mahon (2000) states, art expression, like all forms of expression, is embedded within a cultural context, and as such, art does not transcend culture, but rather expresses cultural norms. For example, within Western culture, art therapy as an individualized form of self-expression is used to focus on the individual that is central to Western culture. Thus originality and personal interpretation are valued within art and 'art', because therapy aims to intensify the voice of the individual as shown in the humanistic theories. This definition of art excludes crafts and decorative directions that are considered 'lower' forms of art. However, within collective cultures, the harmony of crafts' aesthetics can be understood as an expression of the dominant values of collective cultures that stress set roles, static and repeating roles, and social harmony. The craft becomes an 'art therapy' within the context of traditional and collective cultural values.

From this, it is clear that definitions of 'what is art' and 'what is art in art therapy', are themselves culturally constructed and socially contextualized concepts. In other words, art itself has completely different functions within different socio-cultural locations. This contextualized conception of art challenges the universalistic understandings of art on which many art therapy theories and diagnosis are based as shown in the chapters on dynamic theories (Campbell, 1999; Hiscox and Calisch, 1998; Hudson, 1960; Jones, 2003; Mahon, 2000).

The role of the art therapist is to develop methods to reflect on her own cultural assumptions, to learn the client's cultural assumptions from art and books, but most importantly, from the client himself. The therapist makes all of these cultural assumptions about art and therapy, both hers and the client's, manifest and negotiated within the therapy, aiming to combine elements of the therapist's and of the client's understandings.

Evaluation includes analysis of how the cultural differences were negotiated and how they impacted the process and outcomes of the therapy.

Supervision may include assessing the differences between therapist's and client's cultural assumptions and ways that these affect the therapy, as well as addressing ethical issues such as differences in values between client and therapist. Efforts to understand how to make the art most culturally relevant might also be explored.

Research can aim to understand how therapy and art therapy interact with the client's understandings of art and of therapy within different cultures, and on methods that make it culturally appropriate. The concept of the therapist as 'researching' the client's culture, and of the client as research informant, and as owning the cultural knowledge, is central to both research and practice. Another direction might be to understand how different cultures conceptualize art.

Art may be used within research to understand the phenomenological experience of the client's culture. For example, if a client draws a house as a tent, or a house as an apartment block, then these differences are apparent in the art but not in the word. The connection between house and 'home' may be explored by visual rendering, and then by the client or research participant explaining his image. This makes art an excellent method for understanding cultural differences from a phenomenological perspective (Eisner, 1997; Emmison and Smith, 2000; Huss, 2011, 2012b; Knowles and Cole, 2008; Mahon, 2000).

A critique of this theory is that while cultural standpoints are vital for understanding the client and are an important addition to therapy, they are not a theoretical prism in itself. While there is literature on intercultural art therapy, the theoretical understanding of culture is often external and superficial at the level of 'celebrating cultural differences' in terms of external aesthetics or rituals. This is a different form of the level of addressing the deep values and power relations between cultures as expressed through art in terms of what is defined as a problem and what is defined as a solution (Huss, 2007, 2008).

Central concepts exemplified through the case study

Art as a culturally contextualized concept

While art as self-expression of emotions is part of the paradigm of fine art in Western culture, the role of art alters in different cultures, and so art use in therapy is not clear to many people. This needs to be verbally clarified and communicated.

Rina (3B) only agreed to do doodles at the beginning, because in her culture of origin only talented people could draw real images.

Hybrid cultural identity

Culture is hard to define outside of the phenomenological explanation of the client, because most people in global society integrate several cultures in their lives. Often the role of therapy is to integrate conflicting values between different cultures that people live within.

The group as a whole was concerned with female identity and this was discussed on the level of cultural norms that they grew up with. Shoshana (A), a religious woman in the group, was pulled between her need for more time to face infertility treatment and the pressure in her culture to have many children at an early age. The group discussed the Western secular values of having fewer children later, and she leaned on them to help her make a decision to wait.

Power relations on the level of ethnicity, class, and gender

While many clients may be from the working class, as trained professionals therapists are often from a middle-class background, and therefore from a different culture to the client's. Similarly, in some cultures, a male therapist with a female client or vice versa impacts the power relations in the therapy.

While the woman's initial patterns and images can be analysed as stereotypes expressing dissociation from a dynamic stance, they could also be a cultural understanding of art as connected to pattern and decoration rather than to self-expression.

Working the theory: art therapy skills and techniques

Verbal techniques

Culturally sensitive therapists try to learn about their clients' cultural contexts to have an understanding of how problems and solutions are defined, beyond the superficial level of different lifestyles and traditions. At the same time, they also aim to develop awareness about their own cultural values, and to openly discuss these differences between values within the therapy itself. The tension between core values and cultural relativity is complex and needs to be constantly negotiated in supervision, and with the client. Western therapists cannot pretend to be traditional healers, but neither can they ignore their clients' understandings of who should be providing emotional relief – the traditional healer or the educating figure rather than the art therapist outside of the culture. For Western therapists, ethical issues, such as accepting honour killings challenge relativity with basic humanitarian values. Often traditional healers can be included within the therapy so as to integrate or 'translate' the necessary viewpoints. Culturally sensitive therapy aims not to solve these dilemmas, but to activate them and to make them overt within the therapy space.

Another complexity in terms of learning the client's culture is that most people living within global realities are not from a single culture; so a client's culture cannot be learnt as a static entity. Ultimately, the therapist has to become the 'student' of the client, and learn from the client's own self-definition of how the client negotiates his different cultural realities and what his values and understandings of therapy and of problems and solutions are.

Visual techniques

All of the above complexities are doubled for the art therapist, who also has to understand the role of art within the client's culture and according to the client himself. Art is not usually connected to therapy, although it may serve as community embedded therapy. Art is often connected to religion, to talent, to didactic messages, to child development, to cinema, etc., and not to therapy. These understandings have to be negotiated in terms of the therapist's use of art. This may require the art therapist to incorporate new art forms and art places (such as images of gods, or observing a film). Within Western culture art's definition is also constantly changing (e.g. with the shift to digital art making) and so this exploration of what art is doing in therapy has to be undertaken anyway.

Setting

The art therapist can create a culturally contextualized setting, or enable the client to choose the setting (such as incorporating crafts materials, or watching a favourite TV programme, or looking at favourite magazines from the client's culture). Cultural uses of aesthetics and natural visual settings can be transposed rather than the client having to adjust to the art therapist's aesthetic and ideology.

Process

As stated above, culturally sensitive art therapy must first explore the meanings of art for clients, and second, explain the cultural assumptions of how art is used in therapy. The art therapist has to negotiate between the client's uses of art, such as creating charms and rituals with art, and art therapy uses, such as expressing feelings. Once this is clarified, they can then be combined. The negotiation of an art use that is relevant for the client, based on cultural norms, becomes the search, and the creativity of the therapist in learning the new meanings, and in integrating both, bridges and utilizes culture. At the same time, owing to hybrid cultural identity, it could be important for the client to learn Western art forms as a way of understanding the dominant culture.

Art interpretation

The art therapist must be able to self-define her own cultural assumptions about art that are used in interpretation (e.g. that originality is a sign of a strong individual, and conformity a sign of lack of character). A phenomenological stance towards art analysis in which the client is the central analyser enables the client to explain the image in the context of his or her cultural understandings. The considerable dialogue over meanings of the art work makes art a good place to understand the client's culture as expressed in the image. Analysis of unconscious levels, if using a dynamic theory, is very complex for a therapist outside of the culture, and should be undertaken tentatively (Campbell, 1999a; Hiscox and Calisch, 1998; Huss, 2011; 2012b; Kaplan, 2000; Sue, 1996).

Overall skills to practise

- *Ability to define own cultural assumptions concerning art* and concerning therapy.
- *Actively learning about client's culture through books* but also through talking with client as an ongoing process.
- *Learning about the role of therapy and role of art* in the client's culture.
- *Discussing the above and creating a transparent contract* in terms of how both therapist and client understand therapy and art use in the therapy.
- *Assuming a complex hybrid and dynamic understanding of culture* that is based in the client's own explanation rather than text books, or the therapist's own culture.
- *Assuming that art is not universal but has different roles in different cultures.*

Art-based skills to practise

- Discuss or draw the role that art played in your family and in your community and culture. How was creativity defined, who was allowed to be 'artistic' – what role did it play?
- Explore your core assumptions about therapy and about art.
- Explore a problem for you at present and connect it to the cultural assumptions of your family and community.
- Explore cultural expressions in other cultures and the meaning and role of art in that culture, through learning.
- Actively create an art work that incorporates a cultural medium in your culture, such as advertising images, craft forms, digital art forms, or others.

Summary of systemic theories

While there is much discussion of social art therapy contexts in art therapy literature, such as community art, social change, and art in disaster work, or in institutions, the application of social-critical theories still remains marginal within art therapy theory, which is informed by universal psychological and humanistic theories, rather than by social critical theories. The image is often understood as an inherent individualized statement from within the unconscious or conscious layers of the self, decontextualized from social realities, rather than on developing a methodology of creating, discussing, and analysing images through a social critical perspective. This may be because of the historical affinity of art therapy with dynamic and humanistic theories, or due to the struggle of art therapy to become recognized and mainstream as opposed to affiliating with alternative and critical theories (Rubin, 2001).

Indeed, while visual culture, art-based research, and community art have all developed greatly in the last years and in fact have become part of the canon, art therapy seems to have 'missed the boat' of these developments. This is a shame because many art therapy clients are in the public sphere, such as schools, community centres, and health and psychiatric institutions, which have a high representation of marginalized and non-hegemonic social groups. Art therapy clients in the public sector are often facing immigration, poverty, and other social problems. Thus, it is imperative to include a social perspective within art therapy training, as this would be particularly relevant for them. From my experience, while social workers will immediately factor in knowledge of the client's real life situation, they will have more problems working with the phenomenological experiences of the client. Conversely, art therapists will ignore social reality, and escape it by staying within a subjective decontextualized reality. This may be because art therapy is a middle-class profession, and so therapists are less sensitive to the impact of power structures on their own personal lives.

Each of the above systemic empowerment, social change and cultural theories utilize art in a different way, shifting from communication with past roles in the system, with others in the system, with self in terms of lack of power, and with others in terms of taking back power – all within the cultural construction of power and art expression.

Table 13.1 Summary of the role of art interpretation according to social theory

	Systemic	Empowerment	Social change	Intercultural
Setting	Directed by therapist to enhance communication or to shift roles	Art decisions made and interpreted by client as part of empowerment	Setting is within the community and in collaboration with community	Addition of culturally contextualized art practice and locations
Art process	Directed by therapist to create specific change	Directed by client or modulated by therapist to challenge disempowerment behaviours and contents	Outcome oriented and directed in collaboration to create specific effects	Negotiated by client and therapist in terms of cultural norms and understandings
Art product	Used to enhance communication in system, provide new perspectives and illustrate roles	Analysed according to social theories of gender, class, ethnic identity, and power	Utilized to elicit reactions from community and from power holders in media-infused settings	Understood in context of client's culture as explained by client
Therapist role	Active and directive in creating an art process that serves his aims	Negotiating power with client Teaching a social-critical analysis of art and of relationship Connecting to resources in community	To direct the art project to create an empowering art process and effective art product to change standpoints	To understand art and therapy definition in client's culture and to explain therapist's understanding of therapy and of art
Art evaluation	According to its impact in changing the system	According to its empowering impact	According to its empowerment of community and shifting standpoints of others	According to its ability to be effective therapeutically within the client's understanding
Supervision	Focused on methods to change system	Analysing power relationships within supervision and therapy and art products	Mentoring and planning art intervention for social change	Raising cultural issues within the therapy and thinking how to address them together
Research	Researching roles and systems as shown in art Researching effectiveness of art interventions in changing systems	Analysing client case studies according to theories of power Analysing art products in terms of social theory	Evaluating the impact of art on social change	Understanding the roles of art within different cultures. Analysing art therapy process and product through cultural prisms

Table 13.2 Social theories: content, composition, and role of therapist

	Content	Process and composition	Therapist
Systemic	Expression of organizing symbols and understandings in system	Expression of role in system	Shifting roles through creating new compositional organizations
Empowerment	Perceived power and issues of concern	Expression of lack of power or lack of spaces and resources	Analyses according to social meta-theory intensifying clients' own analyses
Social change	Constructed with aim of influencing others	A process of taking back power and defining issues	Directs empowering process and effective end product
Cultural	Content is culturally constructed	Composition and process is culturally constructed	Focus on cultural explanation of content and composition and overt negotiation of client's and therapist's cultural standpoint

Art–settings–populations: pulling it together through theory

Chapter 14

Doing the art

Setting–process–interpretation

As stated in the introduction, many art therapy books are divided according to population, setting, materials, or general introduction, and art activity is derived from these. Another division of art therapy books is for general teaching. However, these do not always break theory or examples down into a set of transparent assumptions about art use (see literature referred to in Introduction). None of these divisions defines the theoretical assumptions behind the art activities suggested. This creates a danger that the question they answer becomes, 'What should I do with the art?' rather than 'How do I address the problem and the solution I have identified through the art, according to the theoretical glasses that I have committed to?'

The claim of this book is that if the theoretical orientation is clear, then the use of art will emerge organically from within it. Section 1 demonstrated in detail how theory leads to different understandings of the role of art within therapy that in turn creates different settings, different use of art materials, different art processes, and different ways of understanding and working with the finished art product. This chapter aims to gather these different understandings into one, providing a bird's eye view of how the art setting, art activity, and the interpretation of the art product all shift according to theory. As stated in the Introduction, the translation of theory into art practice outlined here is only one among many; that of the specific author. It is representative rather than prescriptive. The whole point of this book is that it is the work of each art therapist to start with a theory and to interpret the theory into art activity in relation to a specific client, maybe shifting the theoretical stance when needed.

The chapter will be organized according to three consecutive stages of art practice within art therapy: the setting up of the art materials; the art process; and the interpretation of the art product.

Art setting

The setting up of art materials and the physical organization of the space in which art making happens are subjects much written about in art therapy (Abraham, 2001; Arrington, 2001; Cary and Rubin, 2006; Case and Daley, 1990; Docktor, 1994; Dubowski and Evans, 2011; Gil, 2006; Kalmanowitz and Lloyd, 2005; Liebmann,

1994; Linesch, 1993; Magniant and Freeman, 2004; Malchiodi, 1997, 1999, 2007; Meekums, 2000; Meijer-Degen, 2006; Miller, 1996; Moschino, 2005; Murphy, 2001; Rogers, 2007; Safran, 2002; Spring, 2001; Stepney, 2001; Wadeson, 2000; White, 2007; Zammit, 2001). The setting shifts from one that is closed and encapsulated to one that is open and within the community.

Much of art therapy literature is organized around these definitions of setting (Arrington, 2001; Benson, 1987; Docktor, 1994; Jones, 2005; Kalminowitz and Lloyd, 2005; Kaplan, 2006; Kaye and Bleep, 1997; Kerr and Hoshino, 2008; Landgarten, 2013; Liebmann, 2003; Malchiodi, 1999; Orr, 2007; Riley, 1993; Riley and Malchiodi, 1994; Rubin, 2001; Skaif and Heil, 1988). The art materials can be controlled by the client or by the therapist. There can be full or no art instruction. Materials can also be conceptualized in terms of the spectrum from over- to under-stimulation. Another area of setting that demands consideration is the rules and boundaries of the space, expressed as who chooses the materials, who cleans up afterwards, and decisions of levels of privacy, or exhibition of art works. All of these seemingly mundane or concrete elements become part of the symbolic zone of art practice and have to be conceptualized to reflect the theoretical definition of problem, solution, relationship with therapist, and role of art within the therapy. Another consideration should be whether it is a formal setting, for example, in private spaces, in group rooms, community centres, art centres, or within an institution such as hospital or prison, or in a refugee centre, community green or shopping mall, playground or bench.

The following is an overview of setting according to each theory outlined in this book.

Dynamic theory will translate the central concept of projection within dynamic therapy to the setting, the art room, and art materials. The therapist observes their use by the client, creating multiple projective zones: that of therapeutic relationship, the room, the art materials, and the art activity. This also includes the process, product, and interpretation by client and therapist as well as the final art product. In order to encourage this projective activity, the setting and the art, just like the therapist, will aim to be enclosed and private, but also neutral with a free choice of basic or primary art materials (e.g. clay and paint, rather than cuttings from magazines and stickers).

The projective potential of the materials on the spectrum of controllable versus fluid, colourful versus not colourful, textured versus smooth, merging versus contrasting, pliable versus rigid, regressive versus adult, will all be elements that the client unconsciously chooses to express his inner unconscious but projected world of conflicts, regressions, and defences. Similarly, all parts of the interaction concerning art, such as storage and clean-up, become symbolic projections of regressed and unconscious materials, and are interpreted by the therapist (Case and Daley, 1990; Landgarten, 2013; Naumberg, 1966).

Jungian therapy will aim to include culturally contextualized elements rather than focus on primary materials alone. It will include images of symbols and art products, such as religious pictures, fairy tales, and magazines, that enhance the client's visual engagement with their culture's symbols. The Jungian art setting can become more like an art studio, with an array of different basic but also 'manmade' materials such as small dolls, objects, symbols, and art books – moving away from the dynamic 'blank screen' environment described above.

Art can be exhibited or hung up for further contemplation and analysis of different depictions of archetypes. Art works can be taken to or brought from home in a more fluid way than in an art studio (Edwards, 2001; Furth, 1998; Henley, 2003; Jung, 1974; Wilson, 2001; Wolfgang, 2006).

Object relations may shift the setting to focus on more interactive and playful spaces, using art materials as an illustration and enhancement of interaction between therapist and client. This may include multi-model elements, such as toys and dolls and also include games, places to hang up art materials. and spaces to work together or apart. Privacy, clean-up area, and other considerations will be symbolic zones expressing different types of attachment (Case and Daley 1990; Dalley *et al.*, 1993; Malchiodi, 1998b; Rubin, 1999).

Ego psychology will focus on creating quality art while the covert aim is to enhance positive psychological processes distanced on to the art. For example, sublimation and integration may focus on a more studio-like setting, in which the client can experience new art techniques, and a wide range of quality art products. Art works may be hung up when in progress to enhance reflection but also to find solutions to visible problems, as in an art studio (Ball, 2002; Coleman and Farris-Dufrene, 1996; Heegaard, 2001; Kramer, 1971, 2000; Malchiodi, 1998a; Stepney, 2001; Wadeson, 2000). We see above, that even within the same overall dynamic theory, each sub-theory might shift the setting dramatically according to a specific focus on the theory. These are shown in Figure 14.1.

Humanistic theory is concerned with creating a setting along the spectrum of art as process, art as sensory experience, and art as meaning, in an inseparable and interactive process, which is orchestrated by the client rather than by the therapist. It will translate the basic concepts of self-actualization and authentic communication with self and others in the context of the core condition of unconditional acceptance into an accepting and non-judgemental setting that encourages creative exploration without shame or inhibition. The setting is safe but also flexible, enabling a spectrum of legitimate situations such as areas of privacy, if needed, areas of rest, and areas of stimulation for the client to choose from. There may spaces for joint contemplation of the art product and spaces to leave art in progress (Allen, 1995, 2000; Ball, 2002; Betinsky, 1995; Johnson, 1999; Kapitan, 2003; McNiff, 1998; Moon, 2003; Rogers, 2007; Silverstone, 1993).

Developmental theory, within the overall humanistic stance, will be much more structured, providing and directing art materials according to the developmental needs and challenges of the client as defined by the therapist. Suitability of the materials to the developmental stage, such as level of control, or ability to render detail, or sensory factor, will be carefully considered. For example, a latency-age child may be offered pictures to copy, while a preschool child may be offered finger paints, and an older person with low motor control may be offered easily

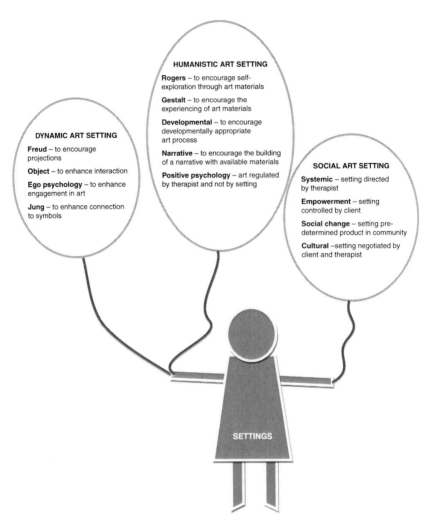

HUMANISTIC ART SETTING

Rogers – to encourage self-exploration through art materials

Gestalt – to encourage the experiencing of art materials

Developmental – to encourage developmentally appropriate art process

Narrative – to encourage the building of a narrative with available materials

Positive psychology – art regulated by therapist and not by setting

DYNAMIC ART SETTING

Freud – to encourage projections

Object – to enhance interaction

Ego psychology – to enhance engagement in art

Jung – to enhance connection to symbols

SOCIAL ART SETTING

Systemic – setting directed by therapist

Empowerment – setting controlled by client

Social change – setting pre-determined product in community

Cultural –setting negotiated by client and therapist

SETTINGS

Figure 14.1 Art therapy settings according to dynamic, humanistic, and social theories

manipulated but 'adult' materials (Magniant and Freeman, 2004; Malchiodi, 1998b; Matthews, 1994; Masten, 2001; Rubin, 2001; Stepney, 2001; Williams and Wood, 1987). The gestalt setting could be similar to the humanistic setting but also include multi-model materials such as music, scarves, and drama props, which encourage sensory engagement. Art work may be presented and hung up to contemplate and there will be room for others to view it (Rhyne, 1991; Robbins, 1994).

Narrative settings suggest art use to create different types of visual narratives. This demands a rich variety of art materials including ready-made elements, tape recorders, collage materials, photography, and film opportunities (Darley and Heath, 2008; Davis and Sheridan, 2010; Frankl, 1985; Save and Nuutinen, 2003; Sclater, 2003). Mind-body settings on the other hand, will focus on the regulative, calming and physical sensations of art materials. CBT and positive psychology will create settings that enable actively changing art works, using materials that enable the client to shift to positive interpretations and visualizations. More linear materials such as crayons and felt tips could be used to map out thought processes and to envisage solutions. Art work may be hung up and photographed, so as to be internalized and to create new versions of past and future issues (Bell and Robbins, 2007; Csikszentmihalyi, 1990; Curl, 2008; De Petrillo and Winner, 2005; Hass-Cohen, 2003; Hass-Cohen and Carr, 2008; Henderson et al., 2007; Rosal, 2001; Sarid and Huss, 2010; Warren, 2008).

Overall, we have seen see that while the dynamic theories focus on creating a projective setting, the humanistic theories focus on a setting that encourages more creative and sensory engagement as a base for generating more meaning and more art. However, it is important to remember that art is not healing in itself; rather the setting of unconditional acceptance is what enables art to be a method to experience the core conditions and ensuing self-actualization that is at the centre of the theory. Similarly, ego psychology or studio art is never a fine art studio, it is a setting for using art through humanistic or through ego psychology theories.

The third set of theories, based on social theories, focus on art as a methodology to reach another aim, such as communication and shifts in roles and standpoints within the system. Thus art is not only unstructured dialogue between self and art and self and therapist, but also a method of communication or interaction with others in the family and group. And unknown others in the community understand that art is an additional methodology used by the therapist to create new perspectives, new symbolic experiences, and new ways of communicating. The setting and materials are therefore used only when needed, and distributed, controlled, and directed by the therapist. The setting is utilized to create a specific experience, such as encouraging roles through joint art activity, or looking for patterns in family or origin, or communicating experience to others (Kerr and Hoshino, 2008, Huss, 2012a, 2013; Riley and Malchiodi, 1994).

Within empowerment settings, the focus is on using art to intensify the participant's voice as a trigger to a verbal explanation. Therefore simple art materials that help to illustrate ideas may be used (Liebmann, 1994). Alternatively, a studio setting enables empowering processes where the client is in charge of all parts of the art experience (Hogan, 1997, 2003; Jones, 2005; Liebmann, 1994). In continuation of this, social change settings will focus, as above, on creating an empowering experience for the creators of the product, but also will regulate the art creating a visually stimulating art product that might influence power holders and change viewpoints. The art setting will be less important than planning a strong conceptual and aesthetic result using the art therapist's art expertise in collaboration with the participant's ideas. The focus will be on creating an art product that is often replicated in the media, and taken out of the art therapy setting where it was created.

From an intercultural perspective, the art therapist could leave the art therapy studio and enter the natural place where art is practised in the community and might suggest culturally familiar art materials and processes (as in a women's craft group, or a religious ceremony, or cultural event) (Huss, 2013). Art materials may be suited to the client's self-defined uses of art, and the cultural understanding of the art therapist of how art can be used for therapy is clarified and exemplified.

Overall, the setting becomes most flexible in social theories often moving into an art studio or a community space. Its aim is not to encapsulate the art activity into a private psychological space but to integrate it into the communal social spaces. This challenges the settings of art therapy by moving into community spaces. At the same time, as already stated in relation to dynamic and humanistic theories, it is important to remember that community art is never fine art, but rather art that aims to change standpoints through a visual medium, rather than to create aesthetic or conceptual innovation. Thus, the social theory is what enables social art therapy.

In sum, the most important point is that once the theoretical aims of the dynamic, humanistic, and social art settings are clear, then they can be symbolically created in every type of physical environment, even if there is not the ideal physical setting. For example, a closed symbolic space in which to practise art dynamically can be created even when working in a hospital moving from bed to bed, with the help of set entry and exit rituals, or warm-up pictures, or creating closed folders of clients' work. Conversely, a humanistic art studio setting can also be created in a hospital with limited materials and lack of calm. Social art projects aim to humanize the system and destigmatize the patients. Similarly, social art can be utilized within individual therapy with a sick child or as a community hospital project by the nurses. The way that the art therapist presents and utilizes the setting is therefore based on the guiding theory rather than on the physical context or type of population or group. These various understandings of settings according to theory are outlined in Figure 14.1.

Art process

After establishing the setting, the next stage of art therapy is the art process within the art therapy. This includes the interaction between client and therapist, and the interaction between client and art materials.

Dynamic theory will employ art in a non-directive way, with the therapist as observer to enable free projection on to art materials and on to the therapist. Process and art product are reflected and interpreted by the therapist in an ongoing way throughout the session (Case and Daley, 1990; Landgarten, 2013). From a Jungian perspective, the focus shifts to encouraging creative engagement with art symbols, as a space in which problems are solved on a preconscious level. Thus, the client is encouraged to engage in art making as a way to solve, and not only to reveal, conflicts, by the therapist who is less interactive in this process between art and client. For example, a teenager might discuss the 'vampire' movies that he/she loves, and the vampire as a shadow archetype can be drawn and developed in relation to the clients own shadow (Edwards, 2001; Fontana, 1993; Henley, 2003; Howard, 2006; Robbins, 1999; Schaverien, 1999).

Conversely, in object relations theories, the therapist will initiate expressive and non-directive playful art making that raises issues of trust, dependency, and individuation in relation to the therapist's role. Difficulties in this interaction enable corrective experiences and are used by the therapist through fresh interactions as well as reflection and reframing of issues. For example, the therapist will suggest helping the client if the client looks lost, and will reflect the client's feelings about being helped (Dalley *et al.*, 1993; Malchiodi, 1998b; Rubin, 1999).

Ego psychology will focus on art projects initiated by the client, but held and actively guided by the therapist who lends her knowledge of materials and art but also her ego abilities as a way to model adaptive processes that could include modulating frustration and self-destruction (Kramer, 1971, 2000; Malchiodi, 1998b; Stepney, 2001; Wadeson, 2000). We see within the dynamic theory, that the therapist shifts from a blank screen, to an ego, to interaction, to enabler of preconscious art work. The therapist uses reflection of these processes and interpretation of them, but also active engagement with art works and with relationships. This includes, within the same theory, shifts from using art to project problems, to using art to search for psychologically adaptive solutions to problems on a preconscious level. Thus, within dynamic theory itself we already have shifts in the spectrum of art psychotherapy to art as therapy.

Humanistic theories will focus on supporting the client through being authentic, respecting, and creating art as core conditions for self-exploration, choosing materials and contents as expressions of authentic self and in an intuitive internal process. The therapist will be a person rather than 'blank screen', using feedback, and his/her own creativity to help the client along the creative path he/she has chosen, offering art knowledge, and suggestions rather than directives. The therapist aims to provide authentic reactions to the art through words or further art making; for example, the therapist might tell the client how moving it was to watch him struggle to find the right colour to express his sadness. These reactions can also be in art, such as the art therapist may see a client very upset and hang up a large page and suggest paints to capture that feeling (Allen, 1995, 2000; Ball, 2002; Betinsky, 1995; Gardner, 1993; Greenberg, 2002; Hansen, 2001; Johnson, 1999; Kapitan, 2003; Lowenfield, 1987; McNiff, 1998; Moon, 2003; Rogers, 2007; Silverstone, 1993).

Gestalt will focus on encouraging the client to connect intensely to emotions in the session through art. The therapist may be active and directive, suggesting ways to intensify the experience such as shifting between art modules, enlarging parts of the art, or changing materials. For example, if a client describes his current problem as conflicts with his boss, but describes it in a distanced manner, then the therapist can suggest depicting this anger visually, or by creating an image of the boss to talk to, or showing how this conflict feels in the body.

All types of interventions are used, but also confrontation may be used to intensify the emotional interaction between client and therapist. Once emotions are expressed they are worked back into the overall gestalt of the client's concerns (Rhyne, 1991; Robbins, 1994).

Developmental art process may actively offer art materials and directives that fit the client's real developmental stage, and also her emotional or 'stuck' developmental stage (Malchiodi, 1998b; Magniant and Freeman, 2004; Masten, 2001; Matthews, 1994; Rubin, 2001; Stepney, 2001; Williams and Wood, 1987). For example, a latency client might be given a game-like activity that also enables expressing former stages through free painting of parts of the game.

Narrative art processes focus on the emerging narrative, around which the client and therapist interact in jointly developing, changing, interpreting, or reframing elements of the existing narrative to the most psychologically enabling form. Client and therapist actively work on the art narrative together, rather than focusing on their relationship. For example, within a narrative about something painful from the past, such as giving up a child to social services, the therapist can actively reframe that this was a brave thing to do as a way to help the child. This can then be added visually to the image, in the form of a symbol or colour (Jones, 2003; Moon, 2008; Riley, 1997).

CBT and positive psychology suggest an active and directive therapist that uses art to direct predefined shifts in cognitions and in experiences of self-regulation (Bell et al., 2007; Csikszentmihalyi, 1990; Curl, 2008; De Petrillo and Winner, 2005; Hass-Cohen, 2003; Hass-Cohen and Carr, 2008; Henderson et al., 2007; Rosal, 2001; Sarid and Huss, 2010).

Systemic theories will have an active and directive therapist aiming to utilize art to create change in a system. It can include concretizing spatial relationships, or using art as a way to express the individual's experience of the system, or using art in a directed way to create a new role; for example, by letting the problem child direct a family art work. The therapist utilizes her own creativity to create a new perspective, or a new experience or to shift standpoints or behaviours through the art use (Huss, 2008; Kerr and Hoshino, 2008; Riley and Malchiodi, 1994).

Empowerment theories will hand the directive power over to the client so that the client experiences power over his own page, symbolizing his own life; in the here and now of the therapy space power is constantly renegotiated by the therapist (Hogan, 1997, 2003; Jones, 2003; Liebmann, 1994). Social action aims to activate the community to define a social need and express it visually in a process that is empowering and also communicative (Huss and Cwikel, 2005, 2011, 2012a; Kaplan, 2006; Kalmanowitz and Lloyd, 2005; Levine and Levine, 2011; Orr, 2007; Shank, 2005; Speiser and Speiser, 2007). From a cultural theory perspective, the art therapist has to actively negotiate between the client's cultural understandings of art, such as creating charms and rituals with art, and the therapist's own understandings of art, such as expressing feelings (Campbell, 1999a; Hiscox and Calisch, 1998).

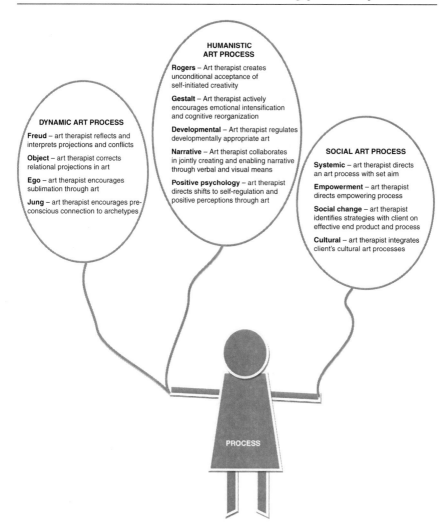

HUMANISTIC ART PROCESS

Rogers – Art therapist creates unconditional acceptance of self-initiated creativity

Gestalt – Art therapist actively encourages emotional intensification and cognitive reorganization

Developmental – Art therapist regulates developmentally appropriate art

Narrative – Art therapist collaborates in jointly creating and enabling narrative through verbal and visual means

Positive psychology – art therapist directs shifts to self-regulation and positive perceptions through art

DYNAMIC ART PROCESS

Freud – art therapist reflects and interprets projections and conflicts

Object – art therapist corrects relational projections in art

Ego – art therapist encourages sublimation through art

Jung – art therapist encourages pre-conscious connection to archetypes

SOCIAL ART PROCESS

Systemic – art therapist directs an art process with set aim

Empowerment – art therapist directs empowering process

Social change – art therapist identifies strategies with client on effective end product and process

Cultural – art therapist integrates client's cultural art processes

PROCESS

Figure 14.2 Process according to dynamic, humanistic, and social theories

The above different understandings of process according to theory are outlined in Figure 14.2.

The final stage in an art therapy session, after creating a setting and creating art activity within the setting, is the reaction to, or interpretation of the art product.

Art interpretation

For dynamic theories, interpretation of art according to defences and childhood conflicts is the analytical prism applied to all components of the therapy, including the verbal interactions with the therapist and the art work. For example, what is the meaning of the client being late to the session, and why are the art materials never enough and why the adult has drawn his mother with long pointed hands? This creates a multiple interpretive zone. Thus, the therapist, the room, the art process, product and reactions to the art process are all symbolic zones for interpretation of defences, conflicts, and childhood fixations. This in effect creates a type of 'hall of mirrors' where everything is bounced back from everything. It is the 'triangle' of art therapy, where the zones of transference projection, and interpretation can occur between the client and therapist, between the client and art work, or between the therapist and art work, and as stated, in relation to the gaps that emerge between them all. This interpretive process is constantly reflected back and interpreted to the client as the central activity of the therapist (Case and Daley, 1990; Kramer, 1996; Naumberg, 1966; Winnicott, 1958). The visual product is interpreted according to the content as expressing the conscious level and the composition as expressing the unconscious level of the client. The unconscious level in dynamic theories are desire and defences; in Jungian theories, they are archetypes within symbols; in object theories they are introjected relationships; and in ego psychology, they include all types of defences of the ego. All are interpreted according to a psychological meta-theory that the therapist knows and the client comes to know and to accept, enabling these contents to be 'conscious' or owned by the client, and this interpretation is what enables him to release the symptoms (Brooke, 1996; Burns, 1972, 1987; Cohen, 1994; Feder and Feder, 1999; Furth, 1998; Silver, 2005; Wilson, 2001).

Humanistic theories by comparison focus on the phenomenological or subjective experience and insight of the client and therapist as the interpretive zone, in accordance with the theory of the client's potential to know himself. This is an ongoing, tentative and intuitive process that occurs on the level of experience rather than only on the level of intellectual understanding (Allen, 1995; Betinsky, 1995; Moon, 2003; Rogers, 2007; Silverstone, 1993). This process occurs through a constant dialogic interaction between art making and art observing or interpreting that is the centre of the therapy. In the more structured developmental theories, these compositional elements of the image express a prior stuck stage, while the content can be developmentally appropriate to the actual stage of the client (Di Leo, 1973; Goodnow, 1977[1926]). Through providing appropriate art activities based on the above analyses, developmental needs can be faced and overcome. Within gestalt orientations, the interpretative level is to experience emotion strongly, and then to be able to integrate it within the overall gestalt of one's life (Rhyne, 1991). Conversely, within CBT and mind-body analyses, the art is only relevant in terms of the outcomes in shifting cognitive-emotional or physiological self-regulative changes. These are blueprinted within the art and can be experienced and measured or evaluated by the client and the therapist.

Systemic analysis is based, as in dynamic theory, on a social meta-theory through which all components of the therapy are analysed. The spatial divisions, relative sizes and interactions between the different elements are understood as expressions of the dynamics of a 'system' as expressed within the spatial and symbolic boundaries of the page. For example, who is left out of a family drawing, who is most central, who is

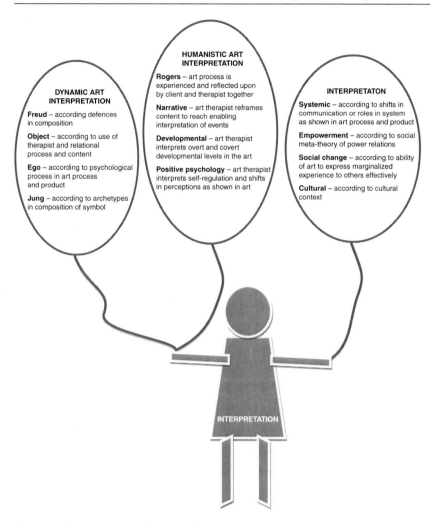

DYNAMIC ART INTERPRETATION

Freud – according defences in composition

Object – according to use of therapist and relational process and content

Ego – according to psychological process in art process and product

Jung – according to archetypes in composition of symbol

HUMANISTIC ART INTERPRETATION

Rogers – art process is experienced and reflected upon by client and therapist together

Narrative – art therapist reframes content to reach enabling interpretation of events

Developmental – art therapist interprets overt and covert developmental levels in the art

Positive psychology – art therapist interprets self-regulation and shifts in perceptions as shown in art

INTERPRETATON

Systemic – according to shifts in communication or roles in system as shown in art process and product

Empowerment – according to social meta-theory of power relations

Social change – according to ability of art to express marginalized experience to others effectively

Cultural – according to cultural context

INTERPRETATION

Figure 14.3 Interpretation of art according to dynamic, humanistic, and social theories

smallest or furthest away, who is next to the client, etc. (Burns and Kaufman, 1972). The art processes and roles taken in group art can also be used to evaluate shifts in roles. Better understanding and new perspectives on the issue will reveal themselves in art products and art processes in the here and now of the therapy. Empowerment theories will analyse art according to gendered, ethnic, and class roles revealed in content and composition of the art. The art therapist may thus actively interpret the image in a different way from that of the client using a social meta-theory (Brington and Lykes, 1996; Hogan, 2003; Jameson, 1991; Jones, 2003; Lippard, 1995; Saulnier, 1996).

Social change analysis is according to the impact of the art process and product on the community making it and on the viewers. Intercultural analyses of art assume that the same compositional elements are not universal but mean different things in different cultures. Analysis is a complex, tentative and constantly evolving dialogue between client and therapist in order to understand the cultural context of assumptions on both sides (Huss, 2011, 2012a; Kalmanowitz and Lloyd, 2005; Levine and Levine, 2011; Orr, 2007; Speiser and Speiser, 2007).

The above different theoretical interpretations of art are outlined in Figure 14.3.

Chapter 15

Individual, family, group, and community

This chapter discusses art use according to the individual, family, group, or community as the context. In accordance with the theory base of this book, this concept is problematic in that it does not specify the theory used within these different settings. Adults, children, groups, communities, and countries can be understood through all of the theories outlined in this book. But as stated throughout the book, the inherent definition of theory is that it is applicable to all types of phenomena, and to different configurations of the phenomena (Cooper, 2008). For example, dynamic theory can be used within a family group and community setting, just as social change theory can be used within an individual setting – as in feminist therapy. In other words, the personal is political, when understood through political theories, and the political is personal, when understood through personal theories. This conceptualization will be outlined below.

Individuals

How can individuals be addressed through social theories? Although Jung is a dynamic theorist, he included cultural context in his theory. Jung's collective unconscious, which is made up of culturally contextualized symbols and archetypes, might be a zone through which individuals address their own problems at a preconscious level. For example, women who have trouble conceiving might be comforted by images of Mary with the Christ child in a church, and this becomes a type of culturally contextualized art therapy, which does not always need to reach the conscious level of talking about it (Edwards, 2001; Furth, 1998; Jung, 1974; Wilson, 2001; Wolfgang, 2006).

Systemic theories conceptualize individual pain as being due to the role of the individual within the system. Often, if the individual changes, then the whole system will have to change. Communicating the pain of a role such as scapegoat to the therapist, understanding it and shifting behaviours to change the role of the individual through the symbolic zone of art processes, becomes a way to intervene systemically through the individual. Art enables other members of the system to be symbolically included in drawings (Huss, 2007, 2008; Kerr and Hoshino, 2008; Riley and Malchiodi, 1994).

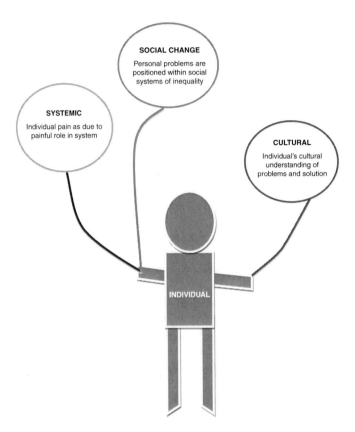

Figure 15.1 Using systemic and social theories with individuals

Empowerment perspectives are often utilized in feminist therapy when working with an individual woman, by positioning personal problems within social systems of inequality. For example, a woman might reach the understanding that, because of oppressive social standpoints, society enabled her husband to be violent to her. She can show and thus resist this violence rather than hide it through art, and also symbolically explore spaces of power and change within her life, by using the blank page to self-define herself. She might join a women's group that works together with her on this, and use art to raise awareness of the issue in society around her (Hogan, 1997; 2003; Jones 2003; Liebmann, 2003).

These uses of systemic and social theories with individuals are outlined in Figure 15.1.

Families

When using dynamic theory with families, the therapist will explore internalized object relations, types of defences, and ego strengths of individual members of the family, in relation to the family of origin and as a parallel process within the current family. The family as a whole system also has defence mechanisms such as displacement on to the scapegoat. Art can be a diagnostic and also concrete space to raise these elements to consciousness in relation to the past and in relation to how they are enacted in the present family. However, art may reveal these unconscious processes to the therapist and to the individual before the family is ready to address them (Riley and Malchiodi, 1994). Art may also be a place to practise more adaptive defences, as a family, such as sublimation instead of violence; or containment and integration of emotions, instead of acting them out in the family; or expression of emotions instead of disengagement. Symbols that are culturally meaningful to the family can become an organizing metaphor that contains the archetypes that the family is dealing with, such as its 'shadow' (Jung, 1974; Kramer, 1971, 2000; Landgarten, 2013; Naumberg, 1966; Riley and Malchiodi, 1994; Robbins, 1999; Rubin, 1999).

Humanistic theories will aim to enable the family to become and to communicate as authentic self-actualized individuals in terms of how they experience the family. Self-expression through art will give space for each individual to define their boundaries and their authentic experience and definition of self-actualization, within the context of the family, and through negotiating the boundaries of the individual within the group – forcing the system to change to enable its members' self-development (e.g. if the mother wants to go out to work). Narrative theories enable the family to create a coherent family narrative of changes that they are experiencing, which can be captured in the art, while CBT and positive psychology can help create images that shift to more positive mentalization of the family and can help to create symbolic processes that teach more adaptive self-regulative behaviours. Developmental theory can observe, through the art, the individual developmental stages of all family members and the developmental stage of the family as a whole; and intervene in accordance with this stage (Allen, 1995, 2000; Ball, 2002; Betinsky, 1995; Gardner, 1993; Greenberg, 2002; Hansen, 2001; Hass-Cohen, 2003; Hills, 2001; Johnson, 1999; Kapitan, 2003; Lowenfield, 1987; McNiff, 1998; Moon, 2003; Riley, 1997; Rogers, 2007; Silverstone, 1993).

In terms of social change theories, art can symbolically redistribute power within the family, in terms of spaces and roles on the page. For example, it lets both adults and children express themselves on the page, and to receive equal 'space' and possibly to bridge different ways of verbal self-expression, enabling adults versus children, or men versus women, or young versus old, to understand each other. In terms of empowerment, by showing the family as individual figures and as a group, as well as the background, or social context within which the family is embedded, art becomes a concrete depiction of family within a broader social system (Butler, 2001; Huss, 2012b; Kalmanowitz and Lloyd, 2005; Kaplan, 2006; Levine and Levine, 2011; Orr, 2007; Shank, 2005; Speiser and Speiser, 2007). In terms of social change, family or members in the family can define and also challenge social norms that are oppressive. They might also understand the family problems as due to social marginalization rather than inherent weakness (Hills, 2001; Hogan, 1997; 2003; Huss, 2005; 2011; 2012a; Kalmanowitz and Lloyd, 2005; Kaplan, 2006; Liebmann, 1996; Levine and Levine, 2011; Orr, 2007; Shank, 2005; Speiser and Speiser, 2007).

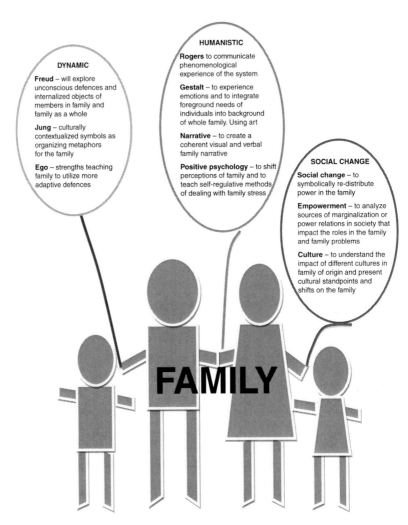

Figure 15.2 Using dynamic, humanistic, and social theories with families

The theories when working with families are outlined in Figure 15.2.

Group work

Within dynamic theories, group art interaction can reveal and re-enact family of origin relationships, with the group leaders as parents and group members regressing to siblings, from an object theory perspective. Art enables these elusive elements to be concretized and confronted in the here and now of the group, and also intensifies the different projective zones. Art in groups helps to capture and to concretize the defences, transferences, and projections that are enacted in both the art processes and the art products, from an ego psychology perspective. Art also encourages integration and sublimation of feelings into art rather than acting out feelings as behaviour within the group. This teaches more effective defences in terms of theories of ego psychology. From a Jungian stance, a group shares joint cultural symbols and can address their hidden archetypes to work on issues of individuals and groups from the same culture (Jung, 1974; Kramer, 1971, 2000; Landgarten, 2013; Naumberg, 1966; Robbins, 1999; Rubin, 1999).

From a humanistic perspective, group work enables members to experience in the present the core conditions of non-judgemental acceptance of all art processes and expressions. Group members, in existential terms, learn to accept others' meanings of art (and through this to accept themselves) and to utilize altruism and empathy towards others and self. In terms of gestalt theories, the cathartic and corrective process of experiencing past feelings in the present with the helps of the group as active witnesses is a central tool. In narrative terms, the art creates safe containers for strong emotions within the group, and help to stress the subjective story of each individual as well as to create a coherent group narrative. The group reactions to the individual's drawn narrative enable the simultaneous production of many new perspectives. Additionally, the group context enables a type of focus group or creation of a group narrative of how people under similar circumstances feel. In terms of mind-body and CBT, the group becomes a place to collectively correct negative cognitions in the behaviour, and in the art work of the group. Art helps to concretize the cognitions, and through directive art activities, the practice of new cognitions and behaviours in the group. Art helps to slow down impulsive or over-stimulated reactions by creating a mediating space. On the other hand, the sensory arousal helps to ignite excitation in those who are depressed or disconnected from their emotions (Allen, 1995; 2000; Ball, 2002; Betinsky, 1995; Gardner, 1993; Greenberg, 2002; Hansen, 2001; Hass-Cohen, 2003; Hills, 2001; Johnson, 1999; Kapitan, 2003; Lowenfield, 1987; McNiff, 1998; Moon, 2003; Riley, 1997; Rogers, 2007; Silverstone, 1993).

Systemic theories are inherent to group practice, by enabling observation within art interaction, the overall roles, coalitions, power relations, and sub-groups within the group as a whole. The group becomes a social microcosm and place to learn new roles through directed behaviour within the symbolic zone of art interaction that occurs in the here and now of the group. In terms of empowerment theories, art enables the group to concretize and then to critically explore power systems and space division. Forms of marginalization may be made concretely visible within the group through art work, and this might be a base for deconstructing them. The group members' joint experience of power systems to which they belong can be explored through art. The empty page may be understood as a zone within which to reclaim power by self-defining its contents. The group can monitor and suggest ways to reclaim power, and art can visualize this. Following on from this, social change systems will use the group first to define the issue to change through art, and second, to work together to create a visual strategy to destabilize power holders or to gain more power (Butler, 2001; Harrington, 2004; Hills, 2001; Hogan, 1997; 2003; Huss, 2007, 2012a, 2013; Kalmanowitz and Lloyd, 2005; Kaplan, 2006; Levine and Levine, 2011; Liebmann, 1994; Orr, 2007; Shank, 2005; Speiser and Speiser, 2007).

Communities

Generally community intervention focuses on assessing and evaluating needs, and on generating the resources and energy of the community to address these needs. This is a cognitive and linear process that has clear aims.

The inclusion of dynamic theoretical perspectives in community work may be very useful; for example, in the types of projections, defences, regressions, and object relations that the community employs. Art helps to access these unconscious elements in a concrete way which may be used within communities to change viewpoints and to raise awareness. From an object relations perspective, community work focuses on relationships, and these are caught within art products.

From a dynamic and object relations perspective, the problem of racism, for example, is that the dominant group members project and displace unwanted internal parts of themselves on to the 'other', by using the defence mechanisms of splitting and displacement (Bhabha, 1994; Freud, 1997; Gay, 1989; Jameson, 1991; Said, 1978; Spivak and Guha, 2003). The solution is to become aware of these parts of the self that are rejected. From a Jungian perspective, symbols can contain community issues, traumas, and hopes. For example, when working with people after a disaster, often it is the visual rendering of religious symbols that help the people to access resilience after trauma, helping mobilize them to solve more immediate problems (Huss 2012a, 2013).

Ego psychology can help to work on creating more effective forms of dealing with pain within the community. For example, the riots that occur in many poor areas in the world are a violent and self-destructive way of expressing the pain of ongoing and deep poverty. If this can be turned into organized resistance, using images and symbols (rather than graffiti with no meaning) then it will be an effective way to sublimate the anger. Art can help to explore the repressed unconscious parts of the self and to reclaim them. From the perspective of ego psychology, communities and countries might solve conflicts through more adaptive defences such as sublimation, humour and integration rather than violence as in wars. This could be within art activities, such as creating a memorial rather than killing additional people. From a Jungian perspective, culture is the place where more primal drives can be released and sublimated (Hartmann, 1964; Jung, 1974).

The inclusion of humanistic values within community work helps to validate all types of individual experience within the community, and to humanize marginalized groups. Art's phenomenological and subjective focus helps to empower and to communicate individual experience within a group context. The use of art within institutionalized communities such as hospitals or prisons, for example, helps to humanize the participants and workers in the institution.

Much of art therapy literature in community settings is based on this humanistic stance of looking at the whole person rather than radically changing society. This connects to changing society, as the right of every person to self-actualize and the need for core conditions may be seen as the basis for demanding equal options for all. The concepts of self-fulfilment and self-actualization often seem to be irrelevant to poor people who are struggling with the first basic needs stages of Maslow's pyramid (Maslow, 1970). However, art becomes a space to regain the right to self-actualize.

From a humanistic perspective, the overall concept of the inherent goodness and uniqueness of all people may be used as a theoretical base to conceptually address racism and marginalization of groups. Art enables the 'other' to be humanized, and to reach the experience of the individual, staying within the phenomenology of the subjective narrative. Narrative theories show how communities as well as individuals need to tell and to retell their collective narrative in order to evolve and to react well to new challenges. Creativity is the natural space within which this important process is enacted, to reignite communication, problem solving, decision making, and to maintain the community's sense of coherence, comprehensibility, and manageability (Kapitan, 2003; Riley, 1997; Rogers, 1995).

A developmental theory will assume that a community (and indeed a country) is constantly developing and maturing, reaching new levels of understanding and different needs. Additionally, the community is made up different developmental stages that each needs different resources. For example, countries with rising levels of old age may need to learn and address the needs of old people. Art can help to express and define the needs of each group, as expressed by the group. This connects to gestalt theories that relate to the ways in which communities as well as individuals need to explore the various components of their shifting needs in relation to the overall gestalt of the community; in other words, the negotiation of specific needs as against the overall backdrop of the community. This may be expressed through symbols of the community as a whole, compared to specific symbols of groups within the community. An example is community theatre where different groups of mixed ages tell their experience of a traumatic community event (Masten, 2001; Rhyne, 1991; Robbins, 1994).

Mind-body theories will address the ways that the community regulates itself; the ways that it can create visualizations of a new future after crises. The practice of art is often an effort to heal mind and body, through mourning, and renewing rituals that include embodied elements, helping to reignite resilience in the community (Antonovsky, 1979; Csikszentmihalyi, 1990; Huss, 2010; Warren, 2008).

If power systems dehumanize marginalized groups, this dehumanization is internalized and the first step is to rehumanize the individual in terms of their own inner experience, so that they can become the subject rather than the object, and can define their own subjective problems, strengths, and dreams.

Community work according to social theories focuses on fighting to create equality. From a systemic perspective, this can be understood in terms of roles within the community (e.g. which sub-group is a scapegoat), and by using art as

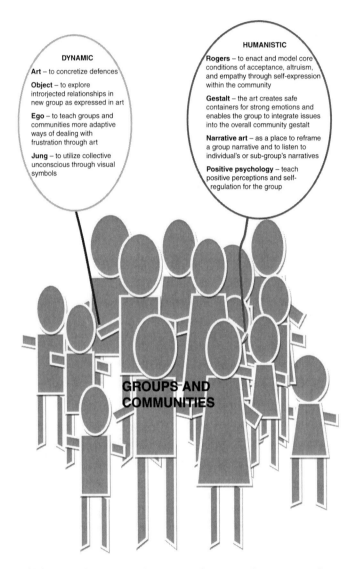

DYNAMIC

Art – to concretize defences

Object – to explore introjected relationships in new group as expressed in art

Ego – to teach groups and communities more adaptive ways of dealing with frustration through art

Jung – to utilize collective unconscious through visual symbols

HUMANISTIC

Rogers – to enact and model core conditions of acceptance, altruism, and empathy through self-expression within the community

Gestalt – the art creates safe containers for strong emotions and enables the group to integrate issues into the overall community gestalt

Narrative art – as a place to reframe a group narrative and to listen to individual's or sub-group's narratives

Positive psychology – teach positive perceptions and self-regulation for the group

GROUPS AND COMMUNITIES

Figure 15.3 Using dynamic and humanistic theories within groups and communities

an arena of self-expression for marginalized groups, which is by definition empowering because no one else is defining them from the outside. Art can be used to communicate within the community. Indeed art was traditionally used within communities to teach and strengthen moral behaviour through street art in areas where people could not read. Within Western culture the values of capitalist consumerist society are also conveyed through images in advertising, as an effective way to change opinions and to thus control people's behaviour.

In terms of social change, art becomes a cheap but effective non-violent media weapon to change standpoints, raise awareness, and advocate redistribution of power. While it is clear how social change settings use social change theories, the ways that individual theories can be used in social change settings are outlined in Figure 15.3.

We have seen that all these theories may be used in all types of 'settings'. The important thing is to learn to utilize all of them when needed, moving from one to the other, or using them simultaneously. Thus, individuals, family groups, and communities can benefit from an integrative and multiple-perspective therapy; art enables enough interactive and reflective space to employ all of these theories together, with dynamic and social insight, reflection, sublimation, and shifts in roles and perceptions, occurring at different times of the therapy, or in a family or group, occurring for different people simultaneously. If the theories outlined in this book are clear to the therapist, then the theoretical orientation of the group is maintained, even as it shifts and is layered. This is a little like riding a bicycle where at the beginning shifts between different skills and perspectives, such as using the breaks, turning the wheels, looking at the surroundings, changing gear, and signalling, are all very complicated. However, with practice shifts between these elements become automatic, and then one can ride in many different directions.

A good example of this can be found in the case study used in the first section of this book of a group of women who are survivors of sexual abuse. Within the group the individual art works revealed the women's deep defences in terms of compositional elements such as encapsulations between objects, levels of control, over-neatness and repetition, anxiety in shading, and using pattern and aesthetics as a way to hide the 'secret' from self and others (see all the visual examples). These compositional and structural levels of the art reveal deep defences such as over-control, rigidity, distancing, dissociation, hiding, and lack of free creativity, within the art work itself (Furth, 1998; Hass-Cohen, 2008; Kramer, 1971). However, the group discussion facilitated direct confrontation of these defences through the art. Gradually, from a humanistic perspective, we see how the women experienced the core conditions of acceptance in the group and created more open combinations of elements, as integrated, connecting, and colourful.

This perspective is also concurrent with CBT and mind-body theories, where the art process becomes an area of reintegrating flexibility and playfulness, and reconnecting between cognition, emotional experience, and physical sensation, which is very important for overcoming traumatic memories. The women created a group narrative of a social situation by sharing their images. From a systemic perspective the group became a corrective family demanding that people shift roles, as expressed within the art (e.g. a woman refusing to take up space on the page). In the end, the women combined all the images into a poster to raise awareness of sexual abuse in the community, turning the same images into a vehicle for social change. Thus, both micro and macro standpoints were combined (Huss, 2009a).

Chapter 16

Deconstructing populations

Much of art therapy literature is organized around art therapy for a specific population (Abraham, 2001; Arrington, 2001; Cary and Rubin, 2006; Case and Daley, 1990; Docktor, 1994; Dubowski and Evans, 2001; Gil, 2006; Kalmanowitz and Lloyd, 2005; Liebmann, 1994; Linesch, 1993; Magniant and Freeman, 2004; Malchiodi, 1997, 1999, 2007; Meekums, 2000; Meijer-Degen, 2006; Milia, 2000; Moschino, 2005; Murphy, 2001; Rogers, 2007; Safran, 2002; Spring, 2001; Stepney, 2001; Wadeson, 2000; White, 2007; Zammit, 2001). This division is problematic in terms of theoretical orientation, because by defining a population as a 'problem' (such as schizophrenia, autism, having behavioural problems, or prison inmates) is often a reduction of the issue, or an expression of the presenting symptom but not the overall issue. This becomes limiting in terms of finding solutions that are based in a theoretical definition of what is a problem and what is a solution and so can lead to a prescriptive rather than encompassing theoretical approach to the intervention.

On a more philosophical level, a definition of population is in itself problematic as it leads to a narrow definition of identity rather than a holistic definition of what is a whole person. Identity is made up of many different 'population' parameters such as the interactive complexity of temperamental characteristics versus social history, or nature versus nurture, that mould each other in the context of a specific developmental stage, to name but a few possible interactions.

Another complexity is that each disability or challenge is different in intensity, and part of a spectrum rather than a 'black or white' entity. Thus, diagnosis versus trait becomes a spectrum rather than a dichotomy. Although diagnosis is important for defining rights and treatments, within therapy we often work with a spectrum. For example, someone may have acute obsessive compulsive disorder (OCD) or general compulsive tendencies, or a person may have physiologically diagnosed hypersensitivity, or be very sensitive; another may be diagnosed as hyperactive, or have high energy and distractibility. Many people have undergone violent or potentially traumatic events to some degree that has left symptoms that they live with. Everyone has experienced different levels of losses and transitions.

While it is important that populations are diagnosed in order to receive the appropriate treatment and to better understand the problem, it is also important

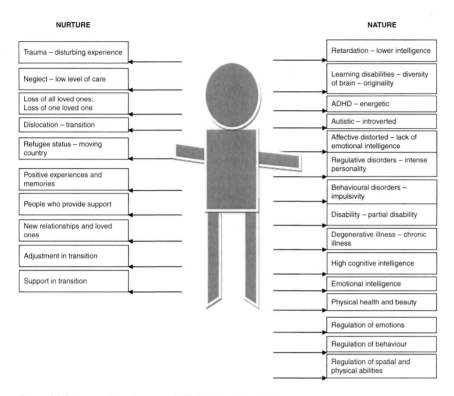

NURTURE

| Trauma – disturbing experience |
| Neglect – low level of care |
| Loss of all loved ones: Loss of one loved one |
| Dislocation – transition |
| Refugee status – moving country |
| Positive experiences and memories |
| People who provide support |
| New relationships and loved ones |
| Adjustment in transition |
| Support in transition |

NATURE

| Retardation – lower intelligence |
| Learning disabilities – diversity of brain – originality |
| ADHD – energetic |
| Autistic – introverted |
| Affective distorted – lack of emotional intelligence |
| Regulative disorders – intense personality |
| Behavioural disorders – impulsivity |
| Disability – partial disability |
| Degenerative illness – chronic illness |
| High cognitive intelligence |
| Emotional intelligence |
| Physical health and beauty |
| Regulation of emotions |
| Regulation of behaviour |
| Regulation of spatial and physical abilities |

Figure 16.1 Interactions between individual and social factors

to understand that all of these elements exist within everyone at different levels. However, the diagnosis is often stated in negative terms, rather than including the interrelated strengths and challenges of the individual such as talents, emotional, spatial, visual or verbal intelligence, or beauty in terms of 'nature', and external resources such as a loving grandmother, supportive community, money, and strong cultural identity or meaning in terms of 'nurture'. These interactions between nature and nurture are dynamic and shifting, as shown in Figure 16.1.

Another complexity relevant to this book is that each theory conceptualizes 'nature' problems. According to dynamic theories, physical, genetic, neurological emotional, and cognitive disabilities or challenges can also be based in problematic early experiences, traumas, or object relations, and the symptoms – somatic or emotional – can be an expression of this repressed experience (e.g. hysterical somatic reactions, or splits and defences as against abusive internalized objects). The solution based on this theory is to raise these inner conflicts to consciousness, to strengthen the ego and to work on a corrective projective relationship. Thus, nature and nurture intermingle, and these problems may also have a psychological component (Berry, 2000; Freud, 1900; Gay, 1989). Somatic emotional and behavioural symptoms can be conceptualized as a type of defence against early pain and conflict. Defences against this pain include distancing from the pain through addictions, dissociation, compulsivity, depression, somatization, acting out the pain (as in behavioural problems) and health problems. The solution is to create a meeting with the original conflict or pain that caused the symptoms and to raise it to consciousness, and understand it.

Art becomes an arena for raising this original pain gradually from a unconscious level to a conscious level. This will help the client to eventually let go of the 'symptom' or the disability that was built as a defence (Case and Daley, 1990; Landgarten, 2013; Naumberg, 1966). Art according to ego psychology helps build more adaptive defences (Kramer, 1971, 2000; Malchiodi, 1998a; Stepney, 2001; Wadeson, 2000).

Object relations will use art to illustrate problematic introjected relationships (Dalley et al., 1993; Robbins, 1999; Rubin, 1999). Jungian theory will engage with visual symbols that contain archetypes that can help to work through the pain and the meaning of the symptoms on a preconscious level (Edwards, 2001; Furth, 1998; Jung, 1974; Wilson, 2001; Wolfgang, 2006). Ego psychology and object relations will claim that even if the symptom is clearly a neurological element, it will make the introjection of relationships and trust in early childhood very difficult. Art therefore becomes a mediating transitional space in which to experience and to internalize trust in a relationship, and to learn to sublimate difficult emotions in an adaptive way (Case and Daley, 1990; Landgarten, 2013).

According to humanistic theory, identity is first and foremost subjective, authentic, individual, and made up of different elements. Thus, if a person has mental, physical, or emotional disability they are part of that person's overall identity but do not define them, and the solution is still to self-actualize their whole individuality through core conditions of unconditional acceptance (Frankl, 1985; Maslow, 1970; Mearns and Thomas, 2007; Rogers, 1993; Yalom, 1994).

Enabling narratives of the role of the disability in the client's life and reintegration of the disability into the overall gestalt are ways to deal with it from a narrative and gestalt perspective. Developmental theories will try to understand how the developmental stage interacts with the client's symptoms. For example, a physically disabled teenager will find it harder to separate from his parents due to his physical dependence on them (Heegaard, 2001; Magniant and Freeman, 2004; Malchiodi, 1998a; Masten, 2001; Matthews, 1994; Stepney, 2001). Conversely, a mind-body neurological perspective will address cognitive-emotional and physical disabilities through medication, and through learning self-regulatory behaviours, as well as through shifting to positive cognitions. Positive psychology will focus on strengths and resources (Antonovsky, 1979; Bryant et al., 2003; Cary and Rubin, 2006; Dryden and Neenan, 2004; Orsillo and Roeme, 2006; Wills, 2008).

According to this perspective, art will reveal the authentic self, and how it can be actualized, in a broader picture beyond diagnosis of pathology. Art enables the articulation of the whole person (Kapitan, 2003; McNiff, 1998; Moon, 2003; Rogers, 2007; Silverstone, 1993). Narrative directions will focus on using art to create a coherent narrative of one's life, which includes the limitations but also the strengths of the individual (Jones, 2003; Moon, 2008; Riley, 1997). Gestalt directions will focus on experiencing difficult emotions and on creating a whole gestalt that incorporates the disability (Rhyne, 1991; Robbins, 1994). Developmental theory will focus on developmental stages that were stuck due to the disability, and on successfully passing the developmental challenges within the symbolic zone of art (Magniant and Freeman, 2004; Malchiodi, 1998a; Masten, 2001; Matthews, 1994; Rubin, 2001; Stepney, 2001; Williams and Wood, 1987). CBT and positive psychology will address negative cognitions due to cognitive and emotional limitations, and focus on strengths and resources to be concretized and expressed within art (Hass-Cohen and Carr, 2008; Henderson *et al.*, 2007; Huss and Sarid, 2011; Rosal, 2001; Warren, 2008).

Systemic theories will address the roles and power relations within social systems that create stigma associated within different types of disability, and that often become the central source of pain for the client. Social change and empowerment will aim to change these internalized roles as well as fighting to change the external systems of disempowerment, which becomes the solution. Concepts such as diversity versus disability self-help and advocacy also become the tools to create a solution (Gladding, 2002; Mernissi, 2003; Minuchin, 1975; Patterson *et al.*, 2009; Piercy *et al.*, 1996). Intercultural theories will focus on the understanding of the issues that the client is facing within his own culture (Al-Krenawi, 2000; Berry, 1990; Cole, 1996; Sue, 1996).

Systemic theories focus on how the art can show and help shift the ways that the disability negatively affects the family system as whole. In terms of empowerment, it shows how lack of spaces and resources but also stigmas towards marginalized and disabled people affect the groups. Systemic theories help by bringing the stigmatized groups a subjective experience, holistic identity, and creativity to counteract this, such as in many disabled theatre and art groups. Art can give voice to marginalized groups that no one wants to deal with, and effectively change standpoints, by humanizing the groups – for themselves and for others. These uses of art to address internal or biological problems are outlined in Figure 16.2.

Just as internal or 'nature' problems are conceptualized differently according to theory, then also the external, or 'nurture' difficulties that define populations (e.g. trauma, displacement, loss, abuse, lack of care) are conceptualized differently by each theory. Dynamic theories will wish to raise the painful experiences of loss or trauma to consciousness through images. Jungian theory will use symbols and archetypes to work through these experiences on a preconscious level. Object relations will understand behaviours such as addiction or criminality as defences against the inner pain of past traumas in abusive or lacking relationships (Berry, 2000; Freud, 1900; Gay, 1989).

Art becomes a way to raise the consciousness of repressed traumatic experiences and relationships (Case and Daley, 1990; Edwards, 2001; Furth, 1998; Landgarten, 2013; Naumberg, 1966; Wilson, 2001; Wolfgang, 2006). Art enables the creation of transitional spaces within which to mourn and to contain traumatic experiences (Dalley *et al.*, 1993; Robbins, 1999; Rubin, 1999). Art enables more flexible defences

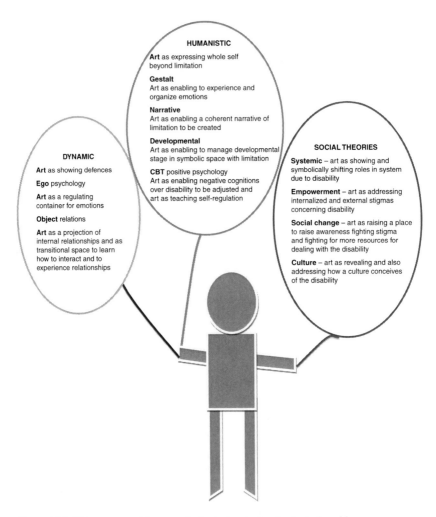

Figure 16.2 Using art to address psychological or 'nature' oriented problems

against the pain of the experiences by connecting to healing symbols and learning to sublimate and symbolically contain emotions. Art enables a re-experience of lost or negative relationships in the symbolic transitional space, and a corrective experience (Kramer, 1971; 2000; Malchiodi, 1998a; Stepney, 2001; Wadeson, 2000).

Conversely, humanistic theories will aim to express the pain of these experiences in a coherent narrative form or to connect to the experience through the emotions in gestalt, or to focus on the whole client and on self-actualization from a humanistic standpoint, within the context of the client's developmental needs at the present time, and the interaction between the event and the developmental challenges

(Frankl, 1985; Heegaard, 2001; Magniant and Freeman, 2004; Malchiodi, 1998a; Maslow, 1970; Masten, 2001; Matthews, 1994; Mearns and Thomas, 2007; Rogers, 1993; Stepney, 2001; Yalom, 1994). Mind-body theories will define traumatic events as an encompassing 'illness' – post traumatic stress disorder (PTSD–) that in effect becomes internalized, and focus on changing cognitions concerning the experience, and on learning self-regulatory behaviours. Positive psychology will focus on the strengths and resources and positive cognitions of the person (Antonovsky, 1979; Bryant et al., 2003; Cary and Rubin, 2006; Dryden and Neenan, 2004; Orsillo and Roeme, 2006; Wills, 2008).

From this viewpoint, art is a place to emotionally and physically experience painful emotions in an authentic way (Kapitan, 2003; McNiff, 1998; Moon, 2003; Rogers, 2007; Silverstone, 1993). From a narrative perspective, art can help to reframe the meanings of the events and to contain them within a coherent narrative. Art enables control, focus, prioritizing, and reframing of difficult experiences (Jones 2003; Moon, 2008; Riley, 1997). From a gestalt perspective, art helps to re-experience painful buried emotions and to integrate them into an overall gestalt (Rhyne, 1991; Robbins, 1994). From a CBT and positive psychology perspective, art helps to find negative mentalization and to concretize positive mentalization of the art work.

Art therefore enables the client to distance emotional intensity and to add an organizational and cognitive focus, thus slowing down processes of reaction, and connecting between emotion-cognition and body, which enable the client to self-regulate reactions. Art also enables the client to encode new memories of past events. Traumatic situations are encoded in the brain first in images, and then turned into words; therefore art helps to access traumatic or disturbing experiences and to integrate them. Art is a holistic activity, and as such reintegrates the physical, mental, and emotional parts that can become disconnected if there is a problem in one area (Hass-Cohen and Carr, 2008; Henderson et al., 2007; Huss and Sarid, 2011; Rosal, 2001; Warren, 2008).

Thus, even if there is neurological as well as traumatic damage, such as after an accident, art from a humanistic perspective can help to address the whole person, and their basic right to authentic self-expression. Art also helps to organize and contain the traumatic accident, by reinstating or reteaching physical (such as fine motor skills), emotional (such as relearning emotions), and cognitive skills (such as learning words again, and defining situations). Art helps to integrate their interaction into a whole, and may also help create visions of resources, and hope for the future.

Systemic theories will focus on negative roles that the experience created within the system and on enabling the system to incorporate loss and change in a positive way. Empowerment and social theories will try to prevent experiences of social violence and lack of care due to marginalization and unequal distribution of resources in society by raising inner awareness and fighting for clients' rights within the specific reality in which they live. This includes negotiating the cultural norms of their social reality (Gladding, 2002; Mernissi, 2003: Minuchin 1975; Patterson *et al.*, 2009; Piercy *et al.*, 1996) and cultural theories will understand how the event is conceptualized and addressed within the culture (Al-Krenawi, 2000; Berry, 1990; Cole, 1996; Sue, 1996).

In terms of external stressors, in general, social theories conceptualize deep and ongoing poverty, as well as wars, violence, and disruptions such as immigration from a position of poverty, as ongoing traumatic events, that might lead to addiction, behavioural problems, and 'internal' problems such as illness, psychiatric, and cognitive disorders. Thus, changing the social system is paramount for healing as well as the nurture level of pain and disability (Alcock, 1997; Bronner, 2011; Foucault, 2000; Freire and Macedo, 1987; Jameson, 1991; Saulnier, 1996; Wandersman and Florin, 2003; Zimmerman, 2000).

In systemic terms, art can first help to deal with the loss of the homeostasis of the system due to change that shifts roles (e.g. if the father dies and the oldest son takes on more responsibility and the mother has to go out to work). Art can help to access how the new system is experienced through intensifying communicative skills and helping people adjust to and incorporate new roles (Huss, 2008; Kerr and Hoshino 2008; Riley and Malchiodi, 1994).

In terms of empowerment, art in a group situation enables the support of others coping with the same social experience of loss, discrimination, or lack of resources. Art makes the problem visible, defining issues, containing intense feelings, and helping people to envisage and think creatively of solutions and strategies for enlisting support to change power holders' standpoints (Hogan, 1997; 2003; Huss, 2012a; Jones, 2003; Liebmann, 1994). In terms of transitions between cultures, art can help with cultural integration. Art is also used in culturally relevant ways to create symbols and ceremonies of transitions and loss (e.g. death or commemoration) because art is a natural way to express the pain, anger, and sadness of loss and trauma (Campbell, 1999a; Hiscox and Calisch, 1998; Huss, 2012b).

At the level of social change, art helps change standpoints, stigmas and conceptualizations of the 'other', and to humanize mechanistic and power imbued values of institutions such as hospitals. For example, use of colours and art work rather than an institutionalized lack of colour and personal touch has been shown to benefit both residents and workers, and to create a less rigid work culture (Huss, 2012b; Kalmanowitz and Lloyd, 2005; Kaye and Bleep, 1997; Levine and Levine, 2011; Mohanty, 2003; Orr, 2007; Speiser and Speiser, 2007; Warren, 2008). The use of art to address social, or 'nurture', problems is outlined in Figure 16.3.

We see above that each theory defines and intervenes in nature and nurture problems differently. From this, the concept of populations is not meaningful outside of a theoretical frame. Similarly, different problems interact from the inside out and from the outside in to create unique combinations of problems within the individual. Internal experiences define outer experiences (e.g a women with retardation is more at risk of sexual abuse) and 'outer' experiences (e.g. long-term abuse or neglect or trauma at an early age) will mould the body and brain. Addiction, anorexia, and others, may be born tendencyies, but are also a reaction to stress. Clearly, in reality, nature and nurture, developmental stages, weaknesses and

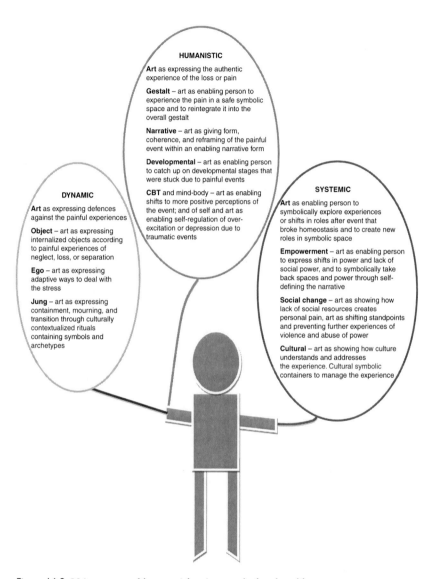

HUMANISTIC

Art as expressing the authentic experience of the loss or pain

Gestalt – art as enabling person to experience the pain in a safe symbolic space and to reintegrate it into the overall gestalt

Narrative – art as giving form, coherence, and reframing of the painful event within an enabling narrative form

Developmental – art as enabling person to catch up on developmental stages that were stuck due to painful events

CBT and mind-body – art as enabling shifts to more positive perceptions of the event; and of self and art as enabling self-regulation of over-excitation or depression due to traumatic events

DYNAMIC

Art as expressing defences against the painful experiences

Object – art as expressing internalized objects according to painful experiences of neglect, loss, or separation

Ego – art as expressing adaptive ways to deal with the stress

Jung – art as expressing containment, mourning, and transition through culturally contextualized rituals containing symbols and archetypes

SYSTEMIC

Art as enabling person to symbolically explore experiences or shifts in roles after event that broke homeostasis and to create new roles in symbolic space

Empowerment – art as enabling person to express shifts in power and lack of social power, and to symbolically take back spaces and power through self-defining the narrative

Social change – art as showing how lack of social resources creates personal pain, art as shifting standpoints and preventing further experiences of violence and abuse of power

Cultural – art as showing how culture understands and addresses the experience. Cultural symbolic containers to manage the experience

Figure 16.3 Using art to address social or 'nurture' related problems

strengths interact in complex ways within the individual and cannot be separated. Thus, the same symptoms or 'population' may look the same but be very different: for example, both hyperactivity and PTSD can create difficulty in concentrating; while long-term deep depression, owing to loss of a loved one, will cause neurological and chemical changes that will react to medication; or attachment deficits in early childhood will create neurological problems in development. In short, the environment permeates our biology, and biology influences environment.

While some theories (such as the neurological or behavioural theories) will state that the source of the symptom is not important, rather addressing the presenting problem, others (such as the dynamic theories) will state that the problem can be solved only when it is clear what its source is.

Most importantly, we see that art in terms of theory does not differentiate between internal or external problems, but instead addresses the problem itself. Dynamic uses of art for lack of ability to connect, because of autistic tendencies or neglect in early childhood, use the symbolic zone to learn to interact and to trust. Humanistic theories, in both nature and nurture situations, maintain focus on art as expressing the whole person – including losses and traumas, disabilities and strengths. Within systemic theories, art shows but also changes the reactions of the system to the stigmatized group.

The above paragraphs aimed to deconstruct the concept of population as a static concept and to reveal its complexity. In order to encompass the interactive definition of population into art therapy, we can think of clients (rather than populations) as a complex and shifting modular collage with interaction between the intra-psychic elements, or 'nature', and inter-psychic elements, or 'nurture', within the same individual at a specific time in her life. Art can physically show this complexity in spatial terms, mapping out internal challenges, or limitations (such as psychiatric or neurological diseases, learning difficulties, temperamental issues, physical disabilities, etc.) and external challenges (such as trauma, cultural transition, poverty, migration, etc.) and showing the relationship between them. This can in turn point to the most pressing or dominant problem, as a starting point, and to a theory that will suggest an art use to address it. This can encourage adaptive, reflexive, interpretive, and creative interpretations of the problem in the context of the whole person and in relation to a specific theoretical stance, which can be adjusted over time. Thus, adhering to a theoretical model for using art, rather than a definition of how to use art with a specific population, can become a way to maintain a complex and tentative understanding of the client.

Overall, this chapter has aimed to demonstrate that if the concept of population is broken down and clients are conceptualized through theories rather than populations, then art helps to deconstruct limiting and stigmatizing definitions of a population, turning all clients first into human beings. The issue remains, however, that how does one choose which theory to use with which population definition first? In the introduction we saw the example of Joseph from the Bible, and the way to choose a theory of intervention was according to the strongest presenting problem at the beginning of therapy. For example, if Joseph is about to lead the people of Israel out of slavery in Egypt, then this is the moment to focus on strengths, problem solving, and visualizations of the future. If Joseph is stuck in his dark pit (maybe symbolizing depression), this is a good moment to delve deeper into the past with dynamic theories (Huss, 2009b). Thus, the strongest presenting problem may direct which theory to use first. For example, a teenager who has a physical disability and is acting up may benefit most from addressing her developmental issues first, and their impact on her disability (e.g. refusal to take medication). This could shift to a family focus, on how to enable her to be a teenager and how the family lives with a disabled teenager. The next theoretical stance could be a strengthening of the self through a humanistic and positive psychology viewpoint, in order to withstand the stress of adolescence. And the final stage may be address the deep attachment issues between her and her mother, on account of the disability, that make it hard for the mother to let go at this stage. Conversely if the family has just moved country, then intercultural issues may be central, and the change in the family roles due to the move (e.g. if the mother has found work but the father is unemployed, making him dependent on the mother financially for the first time), these shifts may be addressed through a systemic stance.

Similarly, in the case study of the group of women who had undergone incest and sexual abuse, we saw the simultaneous use of different theories according to what the women needed at any moment. These included shifts from dynamic use of art to access deep defences against pain, to humanistic uses, to express the whole person and their dreams for the future, to social uses of art to advocate for sexual abuse survivors, and to break the stigma and silence over this issue (see A, B, and C in the introduction to the case study). These could all occur within the same meeting.

An effective way of utilizing the theories to help define the overall internal and external challenges, the developmental stage, and the strengths and stressors of the individual is to create a collage together with the client, of all of the internal and external issues affecting the client at present. They can first be created as individual elements, according to which is most problematic at present, or according to linear history. They can then be organized into a collage in terms of which is the most problematic at present, and the connections between them can be addressed one by one and as a complex whole.

Chapter 17

Evaluation, supervision, and research

Ongoing supervision and evaluation are central components of all types of therapy, and the responsibility of any therapist is to determine how to continue the therapy. It gives the therapist a sense of coherence and direction, and makes him accountable and able to communicate what is happening within the therapy to himself, his peers, and to the client (Ansdell and Pavlicevic, 2001; Gilroy *et al.*, 2012; Malchiodi and Riley, 1996; Moon, 2008). There is always ongoing research in therapy because the client is constantly 're-searched' for by the therapist. The therapist uses different theories in this 'search' to understand the client. Thus, research is vital for practising art therapists just as practice is at the base of all research.

The claim of this chapter, consistent with the rest of the book, is that research, evaluation, and supervision are also defined by the theoretical base of the therapy. The questions of what is being evaluated, how progress is defined and measured, and how the therapist can best move forward in light of this emerge from the theoretical base of how a problem and a solution are defined. For example, while CBT will want concrete evidence of shifts in behaviour to determine that the therapy is effective (Cooper, 2008), dynamic theories assume stages where the client is stuck, or regressed in terms of behaviour, but understands that these regressions are part of the overall process and cannot measure progress outside of the hermeneutic meta-theory (Higdon, 2004). Similarly, systemic theory may evaluate a lack of individuation within a family, while an intercultural theory may understand the concept of individuation as irrelevant to the culture of the client, and so will evaluate different things (Berry, 1990; Sue, 1996). Another example is that while a dynamic approach may evaluate a black image as a sign of depression (Silver, 2005), a social theory may evaluate the same image as a sign of oppression (Huss, 2007, 2008, 2009a). We see that progress and evidence of progress is always based within a research paradigm and epistemology that defines how progress looks. Because of this, different theories demand different types of 'evidence' and the current scientific 'evidence-based' standpoints are not always compatible with all types of therapy, which may be more helped by evidence-informed practice (Waller, 1993). Evidence comes in many forms, such as observing, interviewing, survey filling, experiments, using self-exploration or auto-ethnography, as in a research diary, and other methods.

If we define art not as a universal or physical construct but as a socially constructed phenomenon, the ways it is researched are also socially constructed. Some define art as a path to the unconscious, some as inherently health inducing, others define it as social discourse, and others as an additional methodology in therapy (Hogan, 2003; Huss, 2011, 2012b, Huss and Cwikel, 2007; Lippard, 1995; Mahon, 2000). Thus, art within therapy can only be researched in the context of the role that is attributed to it.

Research methods in the social sciences often divide into quantitative versus qualitative methods. Quantitative methods focus on numerical evidence of a predetermined hypothesis concerning a research question, while qualitative methods focus on subjective, interactive, and context-informed methods of gathering data. While they are often presented as ideologically different, in effect, both quantitative and qualitative methods can be used with all theories, depending on the research question. The analytical prism will always be theory-based (e.g. grounded in theory in qualitative research, or hypothesis in quantitative research) (Gilroy, 2006; Hubberman and Miles, 2002; Wadeson, 2002).

Dynamic theories will access data according to dynamic meta-theory as well as through the client's and therapist's hermeneutic understanding of developments (Kramer, 2000). Humanistic and empowerment theories are more likely to be focused on client's perceptions as central to evaluating the therapy. The the client's subjective evaluation of change is important in humanistic theory, while the observable differences in power are important in empowerment and social change theory (Betinsky, 1995; Hogan, 2003) and can be gathered through qualitative data.

Social change theories focus on changing standpoints, which is measurable through quantitative surveys of communities (Gilroy, 2006; Wadeson, 2002). Mind-body approaches are interested in evidence of physiological change and changes in perceptions and behaviours. These can include biological elements such as stress and hormones, and neurological shifts, which can be measured through experiments. But they can also include interviews which capture shifts in clients' perceptions. CBT (Bell and Robbins, 2007), systemic, and social change are interested in outcome in behaviour or shifts in roles. These theories will analyse data according to shifts in the system that can be observed, measured, or accessed through reporting of those in the system. Empowerment and social change theories will look for shifts in levels of perceived and also real social power (Burns, 1987; Mason, 2002). We see that case study analysis, measurement, surveys, art evaluation, experiments, and interviews, are all relevant data depending on the theoretical stance.

In light of this, art therapy – which as a profession is struggling for recognition, producing evidence for its effectiveness – is concerned that it defines what evidence it is searching for according to what theory the intervention used, rather than following research trends with no connection to theory. For example, while 'scientific' or evidence-based methods are suitable for some theories, they do not capture the hermeneutic and humanistic component of meaning. When evidence that art is effective is used with a theory that is not focused on self-regulation as an aim, it might reduce the therapy to the physical effect of art on the body, as if art were a pill. Indeed, art therapy is so focused on proving effectiveness that it seems to have forgotten the place of interpretive, hermeneutic, and humanistic paradigms within art therapy. Conversely, a refusal to undertake rigorous research or romantic proclamations of art as inherently 'good' for one or as a mystical truth that transcends measurement is also a reduction of art therapy.

To elaborate, we all know that many artists are far from happy or emotionally healthy, and so deduce that art is not 'healing' in itself, outside of the theoretical construct of humanism which provides art as a methodology to reach the authentic self within the 'core conditions' of the art therapy setting and relationship (Rogers, 1993). Humanities education and social science have many rigorous methods of research that are not based on physical or quantitative measuring of data alone. This effort to 'catch the boat' has caused art therapy to miss the boat of the growing 'explosion' in qualitative art-based methods within social science education and humanities, which are more in line with humanistic and empowerment theories. Similarly, there is much concern with creating evidence-based diagnostic art tests, but the use of art as a way for clients to express their understanding of life is not utilized in art therapy, although it is central to art-based research (Eisner, 1997; Foster, 2007; Huss, 2011, 2012b; Knowles and Cole, 2008; Mason, 2002; Pink et al., 2004; Tuhiwai-Smith, 1999).

In sum, research will only provide evidence if the therapy session is understood in the context of the theories that inform it. The research orientation of each theory will be outlined below in terms of evaluation, supervision and research.

Evaluation

Dynamic evaluation is based on the assumption that compositional elements in art, and relational elements in transference, reflect the unconscious conflicts, desires, and defences of the client. Based on this the therapist can evaluate inner conflicts, calcified childhood stages, introjected relationships, attachment styles, ego strengths, and central archetypes and defence mechanisms used by the client. Evaluation will include both the art content and composition, and the gaps in between, as well as the projections on to the therapist, at the level of the transference relationship content and 'composition'. The relationship in terms of the therapist's ability to monitor transferences will also be evaluated in an ongoing form.

Humanistic evaluation will differ from dynamic evaluation in that it will be based on the subjective self-defined experience of the client. The overall sense of undergoing a process, reaching insight, authenticity, self-expression, and clarity and maintaining a non-judgemental authentic connection with the therapist, is an ongoing process that is subjectively evaluated by both therapist and client, and therapist and supervisor, as part of the process of ongoing self-exploration.

Because these processes are lifelong journeys, they do not reach a conclusion, but can terminate when it is felt that they are not needed at present, and when subjective assessment of reduction of symptoms of stress and self-destructive behaviours become part of ongoing and deeper processes of self-actualization. Evaluation of connection to emotions and integration of emotions into an overall gestalt; evaluation of new and better self-narratives; evaluation of shifts to more positive cognitions and more self-regulated behaviour and progress in developmental stages, through successfully completing stuck stages, are all part of the content level of the evaluation (Malchiodi, 1998a; Moon, 2003; Riley 1997; Rogers, 2007; Rubin, 2001). Art works will be used in evaluation in terms of the processes and meanings that they raise and in terms of their ongoing potential for enriched creativity, self-expression, and authenticity. The therapist's ability to provide non-judgemental supportive core conditions will also be evaluated as an ongoing process.

Systemic evaluation will evaluate shifts in roles, power relations, and standpoints of power holders caused by the art, rather than the actual art intervention, because the art is a means to an end (Kerr and Hoshino 2008; Riley and Malchiodi, 1994). Empowerment methods will employ a power-informed meta-theory and evaluate how power is shared with the client and developments in the client's power. Social change evaluates the impact of the process and product on changing standpoints, and returning power to the creators and observers of the art (Hogan, 2003; Liebmann, 1994). Intercultural theories will aim to assess the clients cultural expectations, understanding and evaluation of the therapy within the context of their culture. The assumption is that art will also express socio-cultural attitudes and types of marginalization, as will the relationship, and that art can also fight against them, through making them visible.

Supervision

Dynamic supervision will utilize the supervision relationship as a parallel process to that of the therapy relationship. The supervisor will invest in creating a relationship of containment and safety in order to enable projections and activating interpretation of symbolic content that emerge in the relationship. Because of this use of self and relationship, supervision is central and parallel to the therapy, in that it enables a 'blank screen' for the therapist to project, understand, and unravel the multiple levels of projection – on to both the art and the therapist. This might include using the therapist's art works to understand unconscious elements in the therapy relationship and in the parallel process between therapist and supervisor. The different dynamic meta-theories (Jung, object relations, ego psychology, and others) will be used to understand the behaviour and art works of the client and therapist (Edwards, 2001; Furth, 1998; Henley, 2003; Kramer, 1971; Landgarten, 2013; Naumberg, 1966; Rubin, 1999).

In humanistic supervision, the quality of connection between client and therapist is evaluated in terms of respect, empathy, and authenticity and is monitored and modelled within supervision and reflected within the supervising relationship where the therapist continues to explore his own authenticity and ability to provide non-judgemental enabling core conditions to himself and to the client (Silverstone, 1993). Layers of experiencing emotions, of creating meaning, of reframing negative self-beliefs, and of addressing overall needs in a holistic manner, as the content of the therapy, will be explored with the supervisor. Compared to this, CBT and mind-body evaluations are measured according to clearly defined goals, and evaluated systematically to prove ongoing linear progress. The focus of supervision is how to reach these goals, based on observable shifts in the client's cognitions and behaviour, rather than based on subjective experience. The art enables the client to document these processes and to explore them (Hass-Cohen and Carr, 2008; Rosal, 2001).

Systemic supervision will be based on the supervisor as a mentoring, teaching, and encouraging role model and helper. The relationship will be focused on thinking of methods to create change and on how to implement them in art (Malchiodi and Riley, 1996) within empowerment standpoints. Supervision will therefore be based on the assessment of power relationships within the therapy. Social change uses advice and teamwork to plan social change, and expert art knowledge. The artists or art therapists collaborate with other experts in how to utilize art to create social change. Cultural standpoints will aim to understand clients' and therapists' culture and how they can interact and be negotiated.

Research

Dynamic research can be based on analysing therapeutic interactions according to dynamic meta-theories. This could include descriptive and hermeneutic case studies, where the therapist interprets the client's art making activity and products as well as the projective relationship between them. The holder of the interpretative meta-theory is the therapist. Jungian research will focus on archetypes as manifest across different cultures and symbols, as well as in the client's specific art work. Object relations will focus on the art work as an expression of the relationship with the therapist as projected internalized objects; while ego psychology will try to capture shifts from less adaptive to more adaptive defences in the art work (Edwards, 2001; Furth, 1998; Henley, 2003; Kramer, 1971; Landgarten, 2013; Naumberg, 1966; Rubin, 1999).

In terms of art analyses, because projections of the internal world of the drawer are considered to be evident in compositional elements of art, comparisons of compositional elements of similar populations can teach about their specific defences, or emotional states (Burns, 1987; Silver, 2005; Wilson, 2001). The concept behind these art evaluation tests is that clients cannot self-report on unconscious elements of their personality, or on defence mechanisms used.

As shown throughout the book, these defences and anxieties will be manifest within the compositional elements of the drawings. Thus, if asked to draw basic images such as a house, a tree, or a person, they will project unconscious desires and conflicts, as well as defences, on to the composition of these elements. Purely compositional evaluations address elements such as overall size, location, and line and shading quality. For example a too small drawing of a person could be understood to express depression, while a too large drawing might be narcissistic compensation. As described above, butterflies and other positive elements in a drawing may be a dissociative defence mechanism, expressing an effort to dissociate or distract from a problem. Drawing a person from the opposite sex symbolizes sexual concerns. Large eyes can be understood as paranoia, and poor compositional integration reveals impulsivity. Shading is an expression of anxiety. Large amounts of buttons are analysed as oral fixation. A focus of composition on upper right-hand side expresses optimism, while a focus on lower right-hand side expresses depression. Content elements include bizarreness versus realism, in form and colour, etc. Determinates of mood are analysed according to the assumption that depressed and withdrawn clients will use dark colours, or lack of colour, while impulsive and uncontrolled clients will use strong colours (Brooke, 1996; Burns, 1987; Feder and Feder, 1999; Furth, 1998; Silver, 2005; Wilson, 2001).

Humanistic research will be based on describing rather than interpreting ongoing processes of creative expression. Qualitative methods such as phenomenology, auto-ethnography, narrative methods, and case studies are all suitable for capturing the hermeneutic quality of the experience. The voice of client or therapist may be dominant, or the two may be intertwined, as both interpretations are considered legitimate. The theoretical focus will be on describing the unfolding creativity and resources of the client and the interaction with the therapist, rather than on interpreting it.

Art analyses are also a type of ongoing auto-ethnography, exploring different social and cultural elements as they impact the self (Allen, 1995; 2000; Ball, 2002; Betinsky, 1995; Greenberg, 2002; Kapitan, 2003; Lowenfield, 1987; Moon, 2003, 2008; Rhyne, 1991; Riley, 1997; Robbins, 1994; Rogers, 2007). The use of art as a research method assumes that non-verbal methods can reach more authentic, embodied, and subjective levels of experience, as advocated in art-based research (Eisner, 1997; Huss, 2011, 2012a, 2012b).

Compared to this, research from a developmental perspective will focus on how developmental stages are manifested in art in terms of evolving cognitive and motor processes, such as compositional detail, abstract levels of composition, and ability to create realistic drawings (Goodnow, 1977 [1926]; Horowitz, 2009; Kellogg, 1993). This can also include additional manifestations such as interaction with others and processes of art making (Malchiodi, M, 1998; Rubin, 1999; Williams and Wood, 1987).

CBT will research methods of changing viewpoints through art and on the effectiveness of these methods by measurable behavioural or self-reported shifts in attitudes and behaviours (Huss and Sarid, 2011; Rosal, 2001).

Systemic research and socially based theories evaluate shifts caused by art, rather than the art itself. This includes changes in roles and in experience of roles, and shifts in power relations (Kerr and Hoshino, 2008; Riley and Malchiodi, 1994). In empowerment orientations, the research is participatory because interpretative power is divided between research participants and therapist. Art can concretize these shifts in behaviour and in standpoints.

In art analysis, the family experience can be expressed not only in the content, but also in the compositional elements of family drawings, that will show shifts in role according to size, placement, and overall activity. The compositional elements described, such as size, placement, proximity, intensity, and interaction of different parts of the system with each other, are analysed as a blueprint of a system, rather than as unconscious projections. This type of analysis equates the space of the page with the space within the family and how it is divided between different people according to the drawer's experience of the system (Burns, 1987; Gantt, 2002). As described above, art can concretize shifts that are happening within these systems over time and so evaluate family interventions. Empowerment theories will analyse art according to social meta-theories that explore shifts in roles, resource distribution, and power relations (Hogan, 1997; 2003; Huss, 2007, 2008; Jones, 2003, 2005; Liebmann, 1994). A cultural perspective will analyse art processes, products, and meanings in the context of the cultural assumptions of the drawer about art, therapy, and the contents drawn.

Research into visual culture and art-based methods that aim to understand how social systems and power within them are visualized or depicted in day-to-day life and images is relevant to this stance, and a method for analysing art work (such as analysing images of women in the media in relation to images drawn by female clients). Art can be used to access the phenomenological experience of social systems by marginalized groups, such as minority groups. The assumption is that verbal terms used in academic research and in politics, are defined according to the perspectives of those with power, while images will enable those without power to self-define their experience of social systems afresh. This shifts discourse to the research participant's or client's embodied visual and subjective knowledge, and away from the therapist's knowledge based on abstract, universal, westernized, and often pathologizing, conceptions of clients.

Art, as a spatial medium, helps the client to express relationships between subject and background in new and complex ways, and enables a destabilizing of the hegemonic terminology used in research, inherent to the power relationships between researcher and research participant. As in empowerment therapy, the aim of using art within this type of research is to intensify the interpretive voice of the participant over that of the experts. Thus, the distance between empowerment and arts-based research aims and methods is small and often overlapping. This creates a participatory model of research that is itself a form of empowerment for marginalized and indigenous non-Western groups (Eisner, 1997; Huss, 2013; Levine and Levine, 2011; Tuhiwai-Smith, 1999).

Furthering this idea, the art product as image, film, or other can become the end product of the research, including within it all the visual knowledge found within the research. Indeed, creating art can be defined as a type of research process in itself, which gathers information and experiences of a community or individual, and then presents them visually, to impact those who observe it. A visual end product to research enables many more people to engage with art than just academics who read research papers, and thus becomes a way to influence the world, like social art (Huss, 2010, 2012a).

References

Abraham, R (2001) *When Words Have Lost Their Meaning: Alzheimer's Patients Communicate Through Art*. Portsmouth, UK: Greenwood.

Ainsworth, M (1969) Object relations, dependency and attachment: a theoretical review of the infant–mother relationship. *Child Development*, 40, 969–1015.

Alcock, P (1997) *Understanding Poverty*. London: MacMillan.

Al-Krenawi, A (2000) *Ethno-Psychiatry among the Bedouin-Arab of the Negev*. Tel Aviv: Hakibbutz HaMeuchad.

Allen, P (1995) *Art is a Way of Knowing*. Boston, MA: Shambhala.

Allen, P (2000) Interview with an art therapist who is an artist. *American Journal of Art Therapy*, 39, 7–13.

Allen, T (1988) *Five Essays on Islamic art*. Occidental, CA: Solipsist.

Ansdell, G and Pavlicevic, M (2001) *Beginning Research in the Arts Therapies: A Practical Guide*. London: Jessica Kingsley.

Antonovsky, A (1979) *Health, Stress, and Coping: New Perspectives on Mental and Physical Well-Being*. San Francisco, CA: Jossey-Bass Therapy, 39.

Arrington, B (2001) *Home is where the Art is: An Art Therapy Approach to Family Therapy*. Springfield, IL: Charles C Thomas.

Ball, B (2002) Moments of change in art therapy process. *Arts in Psychotherapy*, 29(2), 99–106.

Bandura, A (1977) *A Social Learning Therapy*. Englewood Cliffs, NJ: Prentice Hall.

Bar-Yoseph, L (2012) *Gestalt Therapy: Advances in Theory and Practice*. London: Routledge.

Belgrad, D (1998) *The Culture of Spontaneity Improvisation and the Arts in Postwar America*. Chicago: University of Chicago Press.

Bell, C E and Robbins, S J (2007) Effect of art production on negative mood: a randomized, controlled trial. *Art Therapy: Journal of the American Art Association*, 24(2), 52–8.

Benson, J (1987) *Working More Creatively with Groups*. London: Tavistock.

Berry, J W (1990) Psychology of acculturation. In Berman, J (ed.) *Nebraska Symposium on Motivation, 1989: Cross-cultural Perspectives*. Lincoln, NE: University of Nebraska Press, 201–34.

Berry, R (2000) *Freud, A Beginner's Guide*. London: Hodder & Stoughton.

Besley, T (2002) Foucault and the turn to narrative therapy. *British Journal of Guidance and Counselling*, 30(2), 125–43.

Betinsky, M (1995) *What do You See? Phenomenology of Therapeutic Art Experience*. London: Jessica Kingsley.

Bhabha, H K (1994) *The Location of Culture*. London: Routledge.

Bowlby, J (1953) *Child Care and the Growth of Love*. London: Penguin.

Bowler, M (1997) Problems with interviewing: experiences with service providers and clients, in Miller, G and Dingwall, R (eds) *Context and Method in Qualitative Research*. London: Basic Books, pp. 66–77.

Brington, C and Lykes, M (1996) *Myths about the Powerless: Contesting Social Inequalities*. Philadelphia, PA: Temple University Press.

Bronner, S (2011) *Critical Theory*. New York: Oxford University Press.

Brooke, S L (1996) *Tools of the Trade: A Therapist's Guide to Art Therapy Assessments*. Springfield, IL: Charles Thomas.

Bryant, R A, Moulds, M L, and Nixon, R V (2003) Cognitive behavior therapy of acute stress disorder: A four-year follow-up. *Behaviour Research and Therapy*, 41(4), 489–94.

Buchalter, S (2009) *Art Therapy Techniques and Applications*. London: Jessica Kingsley.

Burman, E (2007) *Deconstructing Developmental Psychology*. London: Routledge.

Burns, R C (1987) *Kinetic-House-Tree-Person Drawings (KHTP): An Interpretive Manual*. New York: Brunner/Mazel.

Butler, M L (2001) Making waves. *Women's Studies International Forum*, 4(3), 387–99.

Campbell, J (1991) *Creative Mythology: The Masks of God*. New York: Penguin.

Campbell, J (1999a) *Art Therapy, Race and Culture*. Philadelphia, PA: Jessica Kingsley.

Campbell, J (1999b) *Creative Art in Groupwork*. Pampano Beach, FL: Winslow.

Cary, L and Rubin, J (2006) *Expressive and Creative Arts Methods for Trauma Survivors*. Philadelphia, PA: Jessica Kingsley.

Case, C and Daley, T (1990) *Working with Children in Art Therapy*. London: Routledge.

Cohen, E and Gainer, R (1984) *Art is Another Language for Learning*. New York: Schocken Books.

Cohen, M (1994) The status of the Bedouin women in Israel economic and social changes. *Maof Vemeaseh*, 5, 229–37 (Hebrew).

Cole, M (1996) *Cultural Psychology. A Once and Future Discipline*. Cambridge, MA: Harvard University Press.

Coleman, V and Farris-Dufrene, P (1996) *Art Therapy and Psychotherapy Blending Two Therapeutic Approaches*. London: Routledge.

Cooper, M (2008) *Essential Research in Counselling and Psychotherapy*. London: SAGE.

Csikszentmihalyi, M (1990) *Flow: The Psychology of Optimal Experience*. New York: Harper Collins.

Curl, K (2008) Assessing stress reduction as a function of artistic creation and cognitive focus. *Art Therapy: Journal of the American Art Association*, 25(2), 164–9.

Dalley, T, Gabrielle, R, and Terry, K (1993) *Three Voices of Art Therapy*. London and New York: Routledge.

Darley, S and Heath, W (2008) *The Expressive Arts Activity Book: A Resource for Professionals*. Philadelphia, PA: Jessica Kingsley.

Davis, B and Sheridan, L (2010) *Art Psychotherapy and Narrative Therapy: An Account of Practitioner Research*. Dubai: Bentham Science.

DeCarvalho, R (1991) *The Founders of Humanistic Psychology*. New York: Praeger.

De Petrillo, L and Winner, E (2005) Does art improve mood? *Art Therapy: Journal of American Art Therapy Association*, 22(4), 205–12.

Di Leo, J H (1973) *Children's Drawings as Diagnostic Aids*. New York: Brunner & Mazel.

Docktor, D (1994) *Fragile Bones: Art Therapies and Clients with Eating Disorders*. Philadelphia, PA: Jessica Kingsley.

Dryden, W and Neenan, M (2004) *Rational Emotive Behavioral Counselling in Action*. London: SAGE.

Dubowski, J K and Evans, K (2001) *Art Therapy with Children on the Autistic Spectrum: Beyond Words*. London: Jessica Kingsley.

Dwairy, M (2004) Culturally sensitive revision of personality theories and psychotherapeutic approaches: a model of intervention for the collective client. Paper read at the Conference on Psycho-Social Challenges of Indigenous Societies: The Bedouin Perspective, Ben-Gurion University of the Negev.

Edwards, M (2001) Jungian art therapy. In Rubin, J (ed.) *Approaches to Art Therapy*. Philadelphia, PA: Brunner-Routledge.

Eisner, E (1997) The promises and perils of alternative forms of data representation. *Educational Researcher*, 26(6), 4–20.

Elkins, D N (2008) Why humanistic theory lost its power in American psychology. *Journal of Humanistic Psychology*, 25 August, DOI: 10.1177/0022167808323575.

Emmison, M and Smith, P (2000) *Researching the Visual: Images, Objects, Contexts, and Interactions in Social and Cultural Inquiry*. London: SAGE.

Epston, D (1996) *Narrative Therapy in Practice*. New York: Jossey-Bass & Wiley.

Erikson, E H (1993) *Childhood and Society*. New York: Norton.

Fairbairn, W R D (1954) *On Object Relations Therapy of Personality*. New York: Basic Books.

Feder, B and Feder, E (1999) *The Art and Science of Evaluation in the Arts Therapies: How do you Know What's Working?* Springfield, IL: Charles C. Thomas.

Fishler, P H, Sperling, M B, and Carr, A C (1990) Assessment of adult relatedness: a review of empirical findings from object relations and attachment theories. *Journal of Personality Assessment*, 55(3–4), 15–23.

Fontana, D (1993) *The Secret Language of Symbols*. London: Pavilion.

Foster, V (2007) Ways of knowing and showing: imagination and representation in feminist participatory social research. *Journal of Social Work Practice*, 21(3), 15–25.

Foucault, M (2000) The birth of social medicine. In: Faubion, J D (ed.) *Power*, Vol. III of *The Essential Works of Foucault: 1954–84*. New York: New Press.

Frankl, V (1985) *Man's Search for Meaning*. New York: Washington Square Press.

Freire, P and Macedo, D (1987) *Literacy: Reading the Word and the World*. London: Routledge.

Freud, A (1936) *The Ego and the Mechanisms of Defence*. London: Hogarth Press.

Freud, S (1900) *The Interpretation of Dreams*. London: Penguin.

Freud, S (1997) *Writtings on Art and Literature*. Stanford, CA: Stanford University Press.

Furth, G (1998) *The Secret World of Drawings: A Jungian Approach to Art Therapy*. Toronto: Inter City.

Gantt, L (2002) The case for formal art therapy assessments. *Art Therapy: The Journal of the American Art Therapy Association*, 21(1).

Gardner, H (1993) *Multiple Intelligences: The Theory in Practice*. New York: Basic Books.

Gay, P (1989) *The Freud Reader*. London: Penguin.

Gerken, K (2001) Psychological science in a postmodern context. *American Psychologist*, 56(10), 803–13.

Gil, E (2006) *Treating Abused Adolescents*. New York: Guilford.

Gilroy, A (2006) *Art Therapy, Research Evidence-based Practice*. London: SAGE.

Gilroy, A, Tipple, R, and Brown, C (2012) *Assessment in Art Therapy*. London: Routledge.

Gladding, S (2002) *Family Therapy History, Theory and Practice*. Engelwood Cliffs, NJ: Prentice Hall.

Goldstein, E G (1995) *Ego Psychology and Social Work Practice*. London: Simon & Schuster.

Gomez, L (1997) *Object Relations: A Historical Survey*. New York: New York University Press.

Goodnow, J (1977)[1926] *Children's Drawings*. Cambridge, MA: Harvard University Press.

Greenberg, L (2002) *Emotion-Focused Therapy: Coaching Clients to Work Through Their Feelings*. Washington, DC: American Psychologists Association.

Hamilton, M G (1989) A critical review of object relations theory. *American Journal of Psychiatry*, 146, 1552–60.

Handler, L and Thomas, A (2003) *Drawings in Assessment and Psychotherapy: Research and Application*. London: Taylor & Francis.

Hansen, F (2001) *Living the Connection: Spirituality and Art Therapy*. London: Jessica Kingsley.

Harrington, A (2004) *Art and Social Theory: Sociological Arguments in Aesthetics*. London: Polity.

Hartmann, H (1964) *Essays on Ego Psychology*. Oxford: Oxford University Press.

Hass-Cohen, N (2003) Art therapy mind body approaches. *Progress: Family Systems Research and Therapy*, 12, 24–38.

Hass-Cohen, N and Carr, R (2008) *Art Therapy and Clinical Neuroscience*. London: Jessica Kingsley.

Heegaard, M E (2001) *Drawing Together to Develop Self Control*. Minneapolis, MN: Fairview.

Henderson, P, Rosen, D, and Mascaro, N (2007) Empirical study on the healing nature of mandalas. *Psychology of Aesthetics, Creativity, and the Arts*, 1(3), 148–54.

Henley, D (2003) *Claywork in Art Therapy: Plying the Sacred Circle*. London: Jessica Kingsley.

Higdon, J (2004) *From Counselling Skills to Counsellor: A Psychodynamic Approach*. London: MacMillan.

Hills, P (2001) *Modern Art in the USA: Issues and Controversies of the 20th Century*. Upper Saddle River, NJ: Prentice Hall.

Hiscox, A R and Calisch, A C (1998) *Tapestry of Cultural Issues in Art Therapy*. London: Jessica Kingsley.

Hobfoll, S (2001) The influence of culture, community, and the nested-self in the stress process: Advancing Conservation of resources theory. *Applied Psychology: An International Journal*, 50, 337–421.

Hocoy, D (2002) Cultural issues in art therapy theory. *Art Therapy: Journal of the American Art Therapy Association*, 19(4), 141–6.

Hogan, S (1997) *Feminist Approaches to Art Therapy*. London and New York: Routledge.

Hogan, S (2003) *Gender Issues in Art Therapy*. London: Jessica Kingsley.

Hogan, S and Coulter, A M (2014) *The Introductory Guide to Art Therapy*. London: Routledge.

Hooks, B (1992) *Black Looks: Race and Representation*. London: Turnaround.

Horowitz, E G (2009) edited by Eksten, S L. *The Art Therapists' Primer: A Clinical Guide to Writing Assessment, Diagnosis and Treatment*. Springfield, IL: Charles C Thomas.

Howard, S (2006) *Psychodynamic Counselling in a Nutshell*. London: SAGE.

Hubberman, A M and Miles, M B (2002) Reflections and advice. In Hubberman, A M and Miles, M B (eds) *The Qualitative Researcher's Companion*. Thousand Oaks, CA: SAGE, pp. 393–9.

Hudson, F (1960) Pictorial depth perception in African groups. *Journal of Social Psychology*, 52, 183–208.

Huss, E (2007) Symbolic spaces: marginalized Bedouin women's art as self-expression. *Journal of Humanistic Psychology*, 47(3), 306–19.

Huss, E (2008) Shifting spaces and lack of spaces: impoverished Bedouin women's experience of cultural transition through arts-based research. *Visual Anthropology*, 21(1), 58–71.

Huss, E (2009a) A case study of Bedouin women's art in social work: a model of social arts intervention with 'traditional' women negotiating Western cultures. *Social Work Education* (sp. edn: Cultures in Transition), 28(6), 598–616.

Huss, E (2009b) A coat of many colors: towards an integrative model of art therapy. *The Arts in Psychotherapy*, 36(3), 154–60.

Huss, E (2010) Bedouin women's embroidery as female empowerment. In Moon, C (ed.) *Materials and Media in Art Therapy*, London: Routledge, pp. 110–23.

Huss, E (2011) A social-critical reading of indigenous women's art: the use of visual data to 'show' rather than 'tell' of the intersection of different layers of oppression. In Levine, S and Levine, E (eds) *Arts and Social Change*. London: Jessica Kingsley, pp. 1–21.

Huss, E (2012a) Integrating strengths and stressors through combining dynamic phenomenological and social perspectives into art evaluations. *The Arts in Psychotherapy*, 39(5), 451–5.

Huss, E (2012b) *What We See and What We Say: Using Images in Research, Therapy, Empowerment, and Social Change*. London: Routledge.

Huss, E (2013) Bedouin children's experience of growing up in illegal villages versus in townships in Israel as expressed through their art. *Inscape International Journal of Art Therapy*, 18(1), 10–19.

Huss, E and Cwikel, J (2005) Researching creations: applying arts-based research to Bedouin women's drawings. *International Journal of Qualitative Methods*, 4(4), 1–16.

Huss E and Cwikel, J (2007) Houses, swimming pools, and thin blonde women: arts-based research through a critical lens with impoverished Bedouin women in Israel. *Qualitative Inquiry*, 13(7), 960–88.

Huss, E and Cwikel J (2008a) Embodied drawings as expressions of distress among impoverished single Bedouin mothers. *Archives of Women's Mental Health*, 11(2), 137–47.

Huss, E and Cwikel J (2008b) It's hard to be the child of a fish and a butterfly. Creative genograms: bridging objective and subjective experiences. *Arts in Psychotherapy*, 35(2), 171–80.

Huss, E and Magos, M (2013) Relationship between self-actualization and employment for at-risk young unemployed women. *Journal of Education and Work*, 4, 21–34.

Huss, E and Maor, H (2015) Social workers as artists. *Journal of Creative Behavior* (in press).

Huss, E and Sarid, O (2011) Using imagery in health care settings: addressing physical and psychological trauma. *Art Therapy and Healthcare*. New York: Guilford.

Huss, E, Kacen, L, and Hirshen, E (2011) *Researching Creations, Creating Research: Social Methodologies for Researching the Visual: A handbook*. Beer Sheva, Israel: Ben-Gurion.

Huss, E, Elhozayel, E, and Marcus, E (2012a) Art in group work as an anchor for integrating the micro and macro levels of intervention with incest survivors. *Clinical Social Work Journal*, 40, 401–11.

Huss, E, Huttman-Shwartz, O, and Altman, A (2012b) The role of collective symbols as enhancing resilience in children's art. *Arts in Psychotherapy*, 39, 52–9.

Huss, E, Kaufman, R, and Avgar, A (2015) Arts as a vehicle for community building and post-disaster development. *Disasters* (in press).

Huss, E, Sarid O, and Cwikel, J (2010) Using art as a self-regulating tool in a war situation: a model for social workers. *Health and Social Work*, 35(3), 201–11.

Jameson, F (1991) *Postmodernism, or the Cultural Logic of Late Capitalism*. Durham, NC: Duke University Press.

Johnson, D (1999) *Essays on the Creative Arts Therapies*. Springfield, IL: Charles C. Thomas.

Jones, A (2003) *The Feminism and Visual Culture Reader*. London: Routledge.

Jones, P (2005) *The Arts Therapies: A Revolution in Health Care*. New York: Brunner-Routledge.

Joughin, J and Maples, S (2004) *The New Aestheticism*. Manchester: Manchester University Press.

Jung, C G (1974) *Man and his Symbols*. London: Aldus.

Kalmanowitz, D and Lloyd, B (2005) *Art Therapy and Political Violence, with Art, without Illusion*. London: Psychology Press.

Kapitan, L (2003) *Re-enchanting Art Therapy: Transformational Practices for Restoring Creative Vitality*. Springfield, IL: Charles C Thomas.

Kaplan, F (2000) Now and future ethno-cultural issues. *Journal of the American Art Therapy Society*, 19(2), 65–79.

Kaplan, F (2006) *Art Therapy and Social Action*. London: Jessica Kingsley.

Kaye, S and Bleep, M (1997) *Arts and Healthcare*. London: Jessica Kingsley.

Kerr, C and Hoshino, J (2008) *Family Art Therapy: Foundations of Theory and Practice*. London: Routledge.

Kellogg, R (1993) *Analyzing Children's Art*. Palo Alto, CA: Mayfields.

Klein, M (1932) *Boundaries of the Soul*. London: Hogarth.

Knowles, G and Cole, A L (2008) *Handbook of the Arts in Qualitative Research: Perspectives, Methodologies, Examples, and Issues*. Los Angeles, CA: SAGE.

Kramer, E (1971) *Art Therapy with Children*. New York: Schocken.

Kramer, E (2000) *Art as Therapy*. London: Jessica Kingsley.

Kroup, P (1995) *Drawing by Bedouin Children from the Negev in Israel*. Beer Sheva, Israel: Kaye College of Education.

Kvale, S (1992) *Psychology and Postmodernism*. London: SAGE.

Landgarten, H B (2013) *Adult Art Psychotherapy*. London: Routledge.

Lawler, M (2002) Narrative in social research. In May, T (ed.) *Qualitative Research in Action*. London: SAGE, pp. 242–59.

Leary, D (1994) *A History of Psychology*. Cambridge: Cambridge University Press.

Levine, E and Levine, S (2011) *Art in Action*. London: Jessica Kingsley.

Liebmann, M (1994) *Art Therapy with Offenders*. London: Jessica Kingsley.

Liebmann, M (1996) *Arts Approaches to Conflict*. London: Jessica Kingsley.

Liebmann, M (2003) *Art Therapy with Groups*. London: Jessica Kingsley.

Linesch, D J (1993) *Art Therapy with Families in Crisis: Overcoming Resistance through Nonverbal Expression*. London: Routledge.

Lippard, L P (1990) *Mixed Blessings: Art in a Multicultural America*. New York: Pantheon.

Lippard, L P (1995) *The Pink Glass Swan: Selected Feminist Essays on Art*. New York: New Press.

Lowenfield, V (1987) *Creative and Mental Growth*. New York: McMillan.

Magniant, R and Freeman, A (2004) *Art Therapy with Older Adults: A Sourcebook*. Connecticut, IL: Charles C Thomas.

Mahon, M (2000) The visible evidence of cultural producers. *Annual Review of Anthropology*, 29, 467–92.

Malchiodi, C (1997) *Breaking the Silence: Art Therapy With Children From Violent Homes*. Abingdon, UK: Taylor & Francis.

Malchiodi, C (1998a) *Understanding Children's Drawings*. New York: Guilford.

Malchiodi, C (1998b) *Art Therapy with Children*. London: Jessica Kingsley.

Malchiodi, C (1999) *Medical Art Therapy with Adults*. London: Jessica Kingsley.

Malchiodi, C (2007) *Art Therapy Sourcebook*. New York: Mcgraw Hill.

Malchiodi, C (2012) *Art Therapy and Healthcare*. New York: Guilford.

Malchiodi, C and Perry, B (2008) *Creative Interventions with Traumatized Children*. New York: Guilford.

Malchiodi, C and Riley, S (1996) *Supervision and Related Issues*. Chicago: Magnolia Street.

Martin, J and Sugarman, J (2000) Between the modern and the postmodern: the possibility of self and progressive understanding in psychology. *American Psychologist*, 55(4), 397–406.

Maslow, A (1970) *Motivation and Personality*. New York: Harper Collins.

Mason, J (2002) *Qualitative Use of Visual Methods*. London: SAGE.

Masten, A S (2001) Ordinary magic: resilience processes in development. *American Psychologist*, 56, 227–38.

Matthews, J (1994) *Children and Visual Representation: Helping Children to Draw and Paint in Early Childhood*. London: Hodder & Stoughton.

McNiff, S (1998) *Trust the Process: An Artist's Guide to Letting Go*. Boston, MA: Shambhala.

Mearns, D and Thomas, B (2007) *Person Centered Counselling in Action*. London: SAGE.

Meekums, B (2000) *Creative Group Therapy for Women Survivors of Child Sexual Abuse*. London: Jessica Kingsley.

Meijer-Degen, F (2006) *Coping with Loss and Trauma through Art Therapy: Training Manual for Workers in the Field of Assisting Child and Adult Victims of Violence and War When Words Alone Are Not Enough*. Delft, Netherlands: Eburon.

Mernissi, F (2003) The meaning of spatial boundaries. In Lewis, R and Mills, S (eds) *Feminist Postcolonial Theory: A Reader*. Edinburgh: Edinburgh University Press, 489–502.

Milia, D (2000) *Self-mutilation and Art Therapy: Violent Creation*. London: Jessica Kingsley.

Miller, S M (1996) The great chain of poverty explanations. In Øyen, E, Miller, S M and Samad, S A (eds) *Poverty: A Global Review, Handbook of International Poverty Research*. Oslo: Scandinavian University Press.

Minuchin, S (1975) *Families and Family Therapy*. Cambridge, MA: Harvard University Press.

Misiak, H (1973) *Phenomenological, Existential, and Humanistic Psychologies*. New York: Grune & Stratton.

Mitchell, S A (1995) *Freud and Beyond: A History of Modern Psychoanalytic Thought*. New York: Basic.

Mitchell, S A (2003) *Relationality: From Attachment to Intersubjectivity*. Hillsdale, NJ: Analytic.

Mohanty, C T (2003) Under Western eyes: feminist scholarship and colonial discourses. In Lewis, R and Mills, S (eds) *Feminist Postcolonial Theory: A Reader*. Edinburgh: Edinburgh University Press.

Monti, D A, Peterson, M D, Kunkel, C S, Hauck, U K, Pequignot, E, Rhodes, W A, and Brainard, G (2006) A randomized, controlled trial of mindfulness-based art therapy (MBAT) for women with cancer. *Psycho-Oncology*, 15, 363–73.

Moon, B L (2003) *Essentials of Art Therapy Education and Practice*. Springfield, IL: Charles C Thomas.

Moon, B L (2008) *Introduction to Art Therapy: Faith in the Product*. Springfield, IL: Charles C Thomas.

Moon, C H (2002) *Studio Art Therapy*. London: Jessica Kingsley.

Moschino, I (2005) *Drawing the Line: Art Therapy with the Difficult Client*. Hoboken, NJ: Wiley.

Murphy, J (2001) *Therapy with Young Survivors of Sexual Abuse: Lost for Words*. London: Routledge.

Naumberg, M (1966) *Dynamically Oriented Art Therapy*. New York: Grune & Stratton.

Orr, P (2007) Art therapy with children after a disaster: a content analysis. *Arts Psychotherapy*, 34(4), 350–61.

Orsillo, S M and Roeme, L eds (2006) *Acceptance and Mindfulness-based Behavioral Therapies in Practice*. New York: Guilford.

Patterson, J, Williams, L, Edwards, T, Chamow, L and Grauf-Grounds, C (2009) *Essential Skills in Family Therapy* (2nd edn. From First Interview to Termination) New York: Guilford.

Payne, M (2006) *Narrative Therapy*. London: SAGE.

Perls, F S (1992) *Gestalt Therapy Verbatim*. New York: The Center for Gestalt Development.

Perry, B, Pollard, R, Blakely, T, Baker, W, and Vigilante, D (1995) Childhood trauma, the neurobiology of adaptation, and 'use-dependent' development of the brain: how 'states become traits'. *Infant Mental Health Journal*, 16(4), 271–91.

Piercy, F, Sprenkle, D, and Wetchler, J (1996) *Family Therapy: Sourcebook*. New York: Guilford.

Pink, S, Kurti, L and Afonso, A L (eds) (2004) *Working Images: Visual Research and Representation in Ethnography*. London: Routledge.

Pizarro, J (2004) The efficacy of art and writing therapy: increasing positive mental health outcomes and participant retention after exposure to traumatic experience. *Art Therapy: Journal of the American Art Association*, 21(1), 5–12.

Rappaport, L (2008) *Focusing-Oriented Art Therapy: Accessing the Body's Wisdom and Creative Intelligence*. London: Jessica Kingsley.

Rhyne, J (1991) *The Gestalt Art Experience: Patterns that Connect*. Chicago, IL: Magnolia St.

Riley, S (1993) *Group Process Made Visible*. Ann Arbor, MI: Sheridan.

Riley, S (1997) Social constructivism: the narrative approach and clinical art therapy. *Journal of the American Art Therapy Association*, 14(4), 282–4.

Riley, S and Malchiodi, C (1994) *Integrative Approaches to Family Art Therapy*. Chicago, IL: Magnolia St.

Robbins, A (1994) *A Multi-model Approach to Art Therapy*. London: Jessica Kingsley.

Robbins, A (1999) *Therapeutic Presence Bridging Expression and Form*. New York: Routledge.

Robinson, P (1993) *Freud and his Critics*. Berkeley, CA: University of California Press.

Rogers, C (1995) *On Becoming a Person*. Boston, MA: Houghton Mifflin Harcourt.

Rogers, E (2007) *The Art of Grief: The Use of Expressive Arts in a Grief Support Group*. Boca Raton, FL: CRC Press.

Rogers, N (1993) *Expressive Arts as Healing*. Palo Alto, CA: Science & Behavior Books.

Rosal, M (2001) Cognitive behavioral art therapy. In Rubin, J (ed.) *Approaches to Art Therapy*. Philadelphia, PA: Brunner-Routledge, pp. 77–85.

Rose, G (2011) *Visual Methodologies: An Introduction to Researching with Visual Materials*. London: SAGE.

Rubin, J (1999) *Art Therapy: An Introduction*. Philadelphia, PA: Brunner/Mazel.

Rubin, J (2001) *Approaches to Art Therapy*. Philadelphia, PA: Brunner/Mazel, 8–1.

Safran, D S (2002) *Art Therapy and ADHD* London: Jessica Kingsley.

Said, E (1978) *Orientalism*. London: Routledge.

Saleebey, D (1996) *The Strengths Perspective in Social Work Practice*. Boston, MA: Allyn & Bacon.

Sarid, O and Huss, E (2010) Trauma and acute stress disorder: a comparison between cognitive behavioral intervention and art therapy. *The Arts in Psychotherapy*, 37(1), 8–12.

Saulnier, C (1996) *Feminist Theories and Social Work*. New York: Haworth.

Save, I and Nuutinen, K (2003) At the meeting place of word and picture: between art and inquiry. *Qualitative Inquiry*, 9(4), 515–35.

Schaverien, J (1999) *The Revealing Image: Analytical Art Psychotherapy in Theory and in Practice.* London: Routledge.

Schultz, D and Schultz, S (2011) *A History of Modern Psychology*, 8th edn. Boston, MA: Wadsworth Cengage Learning.

Sclater, D (2003) The arts and narrative research. *Qualitative Inquiry*, 9(4), 621–5.

Shank, M (2005) Transforming social justice: redefining the movement: art activism. *Seattle Journal for Social Justice*, 3(2), 531–5.

Silver, R (2005) *Aggression and Depression Assessed through Art.* New York: Brunner-Routledge.

Silverstone, L (1993) *Art Therapy the Person-Centred Way.* Philadelphia, PA: Jessica Kingsley.

Simon, R M edited by Graham, A (2005) *Self-healing through Visual and Verbal Art Therapy.* Philadelphia, PA: Jessica Kingsley.

Skaif, S and Heil, M (1988) *Art Psychotherapy Groups.* London: Routledge.

Skinner, B F (1988) *Beyond Freedom and Dignity.* London: Penguin.

Soja, E W (1989) *Postmodern Geographies: The Reassertion of Space in Social Theory.* London: Verso.

Sokal, M (1984) Gestalt theory in behaviorist America. *American Historical Review*, 89(5), 1240–63.

Speiser, V and Speiser, P (2007) An art approach to working with conflict. *Journal of Humanistic Psychology*, 47(3), 361–7.

Spivak, G C and Guha, R (1988) *Selected Subaltern Studies.* New York: Oxford University Press.

Spring, D (2001) *Image and Mirage: Art Therapy with Dissociative Clients.* Springfield, IL: Charles C Thomas.

Stepney, S A (2001) *Art Therapy with Students at Risk: Introducing Art Therapy into an Alternative Learning Environment for Adolescents.* Springfield, IL: Charles C Thomas.

Steinbach, P (1997) *A Practice Guide to Art Therapy.* New York: Hayworth.

Sue, D (1996) *Theory of Multicultural Counseling and Therapy.* Pacific Grove, CA: Brooks/Cole.

Todd, D (2007) *Against Freud.* Stanford, CA: Stanford University Press.

Tuhiwai-Smith, L (1999) *Decolonizing Methodologies: Research and Indigenous Peoples.* London: Zed.

Valsiner, J (1997) *Culture and the Development of Children's Action: A Theory of Human Development* (2nd ed.) Hoboken, NJ: John Wiley & Sons.

Van der Kolk, B A, Hopper, J, and Osterman, J (2001) Exploring the nature of traumatic memories: combining clinical knowledge with laboratory methods. *Journal of Aggression, Maltreatment and Trauma*, 4(2), 9.

Viney, W and King, B (1998) *A History of Western Psychology.* Boston, MA: Allyn & Bacon.

Wadeson, H (2000) *Art Therapy Practice: Innovative Approaches with Diverse Populations.* Boston, MA: John Wiley & Sons.

Wadeson, H (2002) The anti-assessment devil's advocate. *Art Therapy: Journal of the American Art Therapy Association*, 19, 37–41.

Waller, D (1993) *Group Interactive Art Therapy.* New York: Routledge.

Wandersman, A and Florin, P (2003) Community interventions and effective prevention. *American Psychologist*, 58(6–7), 441–8.

Warren, B (2008) *Using the Creative Arts in Therapy and Healthcare.* London: Routledge.

Weems, C F and Costa, N M (2005) Developmental differences in the expression of childhood anxiety symptoms and fears. *Journal of the American Academy of Child and Adolescent Psychiatry*, 44(7), 656–63.

Wesley, C (2008) *Jung, Folktales, and Psychoanalysis*. Ann Arbor, MI: ProQuest.

White, J (2008) *Sculpting the Heart: Surviving Depression with Art Therapy*. Bloomington, NI: AuthorHouse.

White, M (2007) *Maps of Narrative Practice*. New York: Norton.

Williams, G and Wood, M (1987) *Developmental Art Therapy*. Texas: Pro-Ed.

Wills, T A (2008) *Skills in Cognitive Behavior Therapy*. London: SAGE.

Wilson, L (2001) Symbolism and art therapy. In Rubin, J A (ed.) *Approaches to Art Therapy: Theory and Technique*, Philadelphia, PA: Brunner-Routledge, pp. 40–53.

Winnicott, D W (1958) *Collected Papers, Through Paediatrics to Psychoanalysis*. London: Tavistock.

Winnicott, D W (1991) *Playing and Reality*. London: Routledge.

Wolfgang, G (2006) The ego-psychological fallacy: 'A note on the birth of the meaning out of a symbol'. *Journal of Jungian Theory and Practice*, 7(2), 53–60.

Yalom, I (1994) *The Gift of Therapy*. London: Piatkus.

Zammit, C (2001) The art of healing: a journey through cancer: implications for art therapy. *Art Therapy Journal of the American Art Therapy Association*, 18(1), 27–36.

Zimmerman, M (2000) *Empowerment Theory: Handbook of Community Psychology*. New York: Plenum.

Index

acknowledgement: role and use as concept of Jungian theory 49

action, participatory: role as concept in social theories 111–12

actualization, self-: role and use as concept of humanistic theories 59

Allen, P. 61

analysis, art: role of Jungian theory in supporting 47; use to enable consciousness raising 106

archetypes: role and use as concept of Jungian theory 48–9

art and the arts: significance of psychological theories 1–5; use to address psychological or 'nature' related problems 149–54; use to enable human communication and power reclamation 105–6; *see also* analysis, art; therapy, art

assimilation: role and use as concept of Jungian theory 49

attachment, styles of: role and use as concept of object relations theory 35

attention, media: use of interventions to capture as concept in social theories 112

attunement, reality vs perfect: role and use as concept of object relations theory 35–6

authentic self: role and use as concept of humanistic theories 58

autonomy vs shame: role and use as key stage in development theory 70–1

Avital (case study): biography and art therapy output 16, 17–18; example of art as concretizing solutions to problems and visualizing positive outcomes 85; example of art as connection between right and left brain function 85; example of centrality of concept of core

conditions 58; example of centrality of concept of interaction with others 66; example of centrality of concept of searching for meaning 59; example of centrality of concepts of figure and ground 66; example of concept of regression 27; example of key stage of development generatively vs stagnation 71–2; example of key stage of industry vs inferiority 71; use of art as equalising space in systems 99; use of art as self-regulating activity 84; use of art images to explore family origin 99; use of art symbolic process to capture and change roles 98; use of art to reclaim, use and communicate power 105–6; use of concept of interjected relationships 34–5; use of concept of perfect attunement 35–6; use of concept of projection 34; use of concept of sublimation 41; use of concept of transitional object 36; use of written word to explore power 106

Bowlby, J. 32

brain, functioning of: arts as connection between left and right 85

Butler, M. 110

capture and change, roles of: art as symbolic process of 98

change, social: power of art to nurture 154; *see also* social theories

codification, preverbal: art as concept in disturbing experiences of 84

cognitive behavioural therapy (CBT): application to art therapy 85–6; art interpretation according to 136; art use by communities according to 145, 147;

163; usefulness in assessing supervision 161–2; *see also specific e.g.* development theory; gestalt theory; humanistic theory; narrative theory; positive psychology

humanistic theory: application to art therapy 60–1; art interpretation according to 136; art use by communities according to 144–5; art use by families according to 141; art use by groups according to 143; central concepts 58–9; characteristics and role in art therapy 55; characteristics of evaluation of art therapy utilising 57; context and macro applications 56; critique of 57–8; interpretation of art settings according to 129; interpretation of therapy processes according to 133; overview of content, composition and role of therapist 87–91; role of art and art therapist according to 56–7; role of therapy supervision and research utilising 57; significance for art and therapy 5; summary of role in relation to art therapy 53–4

identification, research problem: role and use as key stage and concept in narrative theory 78

identity vs role confusion: role and use as key stage in development theory 71

identity, hybrid: role as concept in cultural theories 119

images, art: use to explore family origin 98

individuals: art use by according to empowerment theory 140; art use by according to Jungian theory 139; art use by according to social theories 139–40; art use by according to systemic theories 139–40

industry vs inferiority: role and use as key stage in development theory 71

initiative vs guilt: role and use as key stage in development theory 71

insight, personal: role and use as concept of humanistic theories 59

integration: role and use as concept of ego psychology theory 41

integrity (ego integrity) vs despair: role and use as key stage in development theory 72

interaction, human: role and use as concept of gestalt theory 66

interpretation: personal vs social as concept in empowerment theories 105; role and use as concept of psychodynamic theory 27

interpretation, art: according to CBT 139; according to ego psychology 139; according to humanistic theory 139; according to Jungian theory 139; according to psychodynamic theory 138–9; according to social change theory 139–40; according to systemic theory 139–40; role of cultural theories in supporting 121; role of cultural theories in supporting 123; role of development theory in supporting 73; role of ego psychology in supporting 42; role of empowerment theories in supporting 107–8; role of humanistic theories in supporting 61; role of narrative theory in supporting 79; role of object relations theory in supporting 37; role of positive psychology in supporting 86; role of social theories in supporting 114; role of systemic theory in supporting 99

interventions, multi-model: use as concept in social theories 112

intimacy vs loneliness: role and use as key stage in development theory 71

Jung, C. 21, 61

Jungian theory: application to art therapy 46–8; art interpretation according to 136; art use by communities according to 144; art use by groups according to 143; art use by individuals according to 139; central concepts 48–9; characteristics of evaluation of art therapy utilising 47; context and macro theories 44–5; critique of 48; interpretation of art settings according to 128–9; interpretation of therapy processes according to 132–3; role of art and art therapist according to 45–6; role of therapy supervision and research utilising 47–8; summary of role in relation to art therapy 44

Klein, M. 32

Kramer, E. 40

libidinal energy theory (Freud) 5

Mahon, M. 117

theories in supporting 60; role of Jungian
theory in supporting 46; role of narrative
theory in supporting 79; role of object
relations theory in supporting 37; role
of positive psychology in supporting
86; role of psychodynamic theory in
supporting 29; role of social theories in
supporting 113; role of systemic theory
in supporting 99

Sharon (case study): art as expression of
how individual uses the 'system' 99; art
as proverbial codification of disturbing
experiences 84; biography and art
therapy output 12, 14–15, 16; centrality
of concept of authentic self 58; centrality
of concept of layers of neurosis 65;
concept of confronting personal pain 78;
transference and counter-transference 27;
use of arts as self-regulating activity 84;
use of concept of attachment styles 35

Shoshana (case study): art as concretizing
solutions to problems and visualizing
positive outcomes 85; biography and
art therapy output 8–10, 11; centrality
of concept of immediate experience
65; centrality of concept of interaction
with others 66; centrality of concept
of pyramid of needs 59; centrality
of concept of self-actualization 59;
challenge of hybrid cultural identity
119; concept of verbal vs visual
problems in research 77; key stage of
autonomy vs shame and doubt 70–1;
key stage of development vs stagnation
71–2; key stage of ego integrity vs
despair 72; key stage of research
problem exploration and identification
78; key stage of research reconstruction,
negotiation and evolution 78; key stages
of identity vs confusion and intimacy
vs loneliness 71; key stages of identity
vs confusion and intimacy vs loneliness
71; of use of concept of collective
unconscious 48; of use of concepts
of familiarization, acknowledgement,
assimilation and disposal 49; use of
arts as self-regulating activity 84;
use of concept of symbolization
and sublimation 41; use of group to
challenge social stands 106

skills, art therapy see techniques, art therapy
social theories: application to art therapy
112–14; art interpretation according to

138; art use by communities according
to 145–7; art use by families according
to 141; art use by individuals according
to social theories 139–40; central
concepts 111–12; characteristics and role
in art therapy 109; context and micro
applications 109–10; critique of 111;
overview of content, composition and role
of therapist 122–4; problem for therapy
of conceptualisations of 154; role of art
and art therapist according to 110; role of
therapy supervision and research utilising
110–11; significance of theoretical base for
158, 159

space: art as concept of equalizing 97
space, transitional: role and use as concept
of object relations theory 36
spaces, art see settings, art therapy
Spivak, G. 103
strategies, planning and communication:
role as concept in cultural theories 118–
19; role as concept in social theories 112
sublimation: role and use as concept of ego
psychology theory 41
supervision, art therapy: role humanistic
theories in supporting 57; role of CBT
in supporting 83–4; role of cultural
theories in supporting 118; role of
development theory in supporting 69;
role of ego psychology in supporting
40–1; role of empowerment theories
in supporting 104–5; role of gestalt in
supporting 64–5; role of Jungian theory
in supporting art therapy 47; role of
narrative theory in supporting 77; role of
object relations theory in supporting 34;
role of positive psychology in supporting
83–4; role of psychodynamic theory
supporting 26; role of social theories
supporting 110–11; role of systemic
theory supporting 96; significance in
psychodynamic theory 26; significance of
theoretical base for art therapy 158–60,
161–2; usefulness of CBT in assessing
163; usefulness of humanistic theories in
assessing 161–2; usefulness of systemic
theories in assessing 162
symbolization: role and use as concept of
ego psychology theory 41
symbols: role and use as concept of Jungian
theory 48
'system,' the: art as expression of how
individual experiences 97